Mental Health Nursing

To the memory of my mother Ruby Miriam Watkins who taught me about caring

Senior commissioning editor: Mary Seager
Development editor: Caroline Savage
Production controller: Anthony Read
Desk editor: Angela Davies
Cover designer: Fred Rose

Mental Health Nursing:

the art of compassionate care

Peter Watkins M.Ed., R.N.T., Dip N., Dip Hum. Psych., R.M.N.
Mental Health Nurse Care Manager with the Assertive Outreach Service, Local Health Partnerships NHS Trust Ipswich
Formerly Senior Lecturer in Mental Health Nursing at Suffolk College, Ipswich, UK

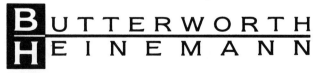

BUTTERWORTH
HEINEMANN

OXFORD AUCKLAND BOSTON JOHANNESBURG MELBOURNE NEW DELHI

Butterworth-Heinemann
Robert Stevenson House, 1-3 Baxter's Place
Leith Walk, Edinburgh EH1 3AF

First published 2001
Reprinted 2002

British Library Cataloguing in Publication Data
Watkins, Peter
  Mental health nursing: the art of compassionate care
  1. Psychiatric nursing
  I. Title
  610.7′368

Library of Congress Cataloging in Publication Data
Watkins, Peter, 1939–
  Mental health nursing: the art of compassionate care / Peter Watkins.
  p. cm.
  Includes bibliographical references and index.
  ISBN 0 7506 4119 3
  1. Psychiatric nursing   I. Title.
RC440.W36 2000
610.73′68–dc21   00–057172

ISBN 0 7506 4119 3

Printed and bound in Great Britain by Biddles Ltd, *www.biddles.co.uk*

ELSEVIER
SCIENCE
your source for books,
journals and multimedia
in the health sciences
www.elsevierhealth.com

Contents

Part 4
Personal management   187

Introduction

This book is a reflection on mental health care and, in particular, mental health nursing. At its core is an exploration of the helping relationship and the caring process. During the 35 years that I have been a psychiatric nurse I have come to believe strongly in compassionate care as the mainspring of recovery. Unfortunately, over the last few decades the compassionate care of deeply troubled people has come to be valued less than the psycho-technologies. These days everyone wants to be a therapist! You will find very little 'therapy' in this book. What you will find is an exploration of the nature of restorative care in the context of the mental health services.

Most of my experience over the years has been with people who have struggled not only with their own disabling distress, but also with the oppression and stigma that comes with enduring mental health problems. Many of them have been inspiring examples of the indomitable nature of the human spirit when faced with continuing anguish and adversity. I often ask myself how I would cope with the afflictions and deprivation that many users of the mental health services survive and recover from. What sustains the human spirit through such troubled states of mind, when distress is so enveloping that everyday living becomes difficult, if not impossible, is the empathic and compassionate presence of another who can be a caretaker of hope. You cannot work in an enabling way with people unless you believe in the potential of everyone to grow and change in the direction of becoming fully functioning people. People who are able to manage the challenges and opportunities of living more effectively, discover a personal identity that is not circumscribed by vulnerability and disability and recover an ordinary life that offers a measure of the joys and satisfactions we all seek. In making this point, I am not suggesting that the recovery pathway is one that is easily found or taken. Many people get stuck in a therapeutic system that often sees people as prisoners of misfortune, a perspective from which the best one can hope for is to mitigate recurrent distress with drugs and support.

Throughout the book I have tried to avoid the conventional language of psychiatry, which can be mystifying and excluding. Biomedical psychiatry has, over the years, erroneously acquired the status of a scientific truth, a status that confers enormous power on those who hold this knowledge. To claim an empirical understanding of human vulnerability to disabling distress simply from the biomedical perspective is arrogant nonsense. As individuals we have a uniqueness and complexity that defies such a structuralist approach. A similar charge can be levelled against psychological models, which locate the cause of distress in the inner world, largely ignoring the social context in which people live their lives. Mental health nursing takes a more holistic, person-centred view of human distress, seeing the client as the only true expert, the only person who has knowledge of the lived experience that has influenced their way of being in the world. As nurses, we have the privileged role of standing alongside people in the landscape of their lives. If we can listen empathically enough, we can witness the journey that has brought them to their present place and offer companionship, comfort and encouragement to continue their journey along a more sustaining path.

The first part of the book is an exploration of the experience of severe and disabling distress, the recovery process and the values that underpin a person-centred approach to therapeutic care. Part 2 examines the nature of the working alliance between people who use the mental health services and mental health professionals. The third part of the book goes beyond the working alliance to consider the various forms the intentional use of self can take in aiding the process of recovery. In the final section, the focus is on the interface between the professional and personal. It argues that the art of compassionate care depends on a commitment to personal development as an integral part of our growth as mental health professionals. If we are to give of our best, we have a responsibility to sustain our capacity to care compassionately through recognizing and respecting our own needs.

Significant learning is a process not just of engagement and assimilation, but of integration. Making new learning a part of ourselves, part of the way we think, feel and act involves an interaction with the material not just cognitively, but affectively and behaviourally. The self-enquiry exercises that form part of the text are offered as a structured invitation to interact with the key themes. The personal narratives that appear in the book are largely authentic though, of course, altered to protect anonymity. It has been the experience of disabling distress of people I have worked with over the years that has taught me most and it is the glow of their testimonies that I hope illuminates the text.

The book has been written as a foundation for good practice in mental health care. It has been written with mental health nurses in mind, simply because I am a nurse. Yet I am very conscious of the shared skill base of the various professional disciplines working in the mental health services and of the generic nature of practice in some multidisciplinary teams. Therefore, much of the book will have a direct relevance to the work of social workers, occupational therapists, psychologists, arts therapists, psychiatrists and to mental health support workers, who have come to play an increasingly important role within mental health services. I have intentionally used the more generic term mental health practitioner extensively in the text and I hope no one will feel excluded where a specific reference to mental health nurses has been used.

The key theoretical influences on my thinking will be readily apparent, even from a cursory glance at the text. The ideas of Carl Rogers, John Heron and Gerard Egan have been sustaining for me, both philosophically and practically, throughout much of my career. What links them is their humanistic orientation and it is in the fertile soil of humanistic psychology that the contents of this book have their deepest roots. But it is not just the work of these innovative thinkers that has informed this text. It has been my good fortune to work with many gifted educationalists and clinicians whose teaching and practice has exemplified compassionate care and I am conscious that something of their work has been distilled into the pages of this book.

My heartfelt thanks to those close to me for their patience, encouragement and support throughout the book's long 'gestation'. I owe a special debt of gratitude to my partner Ann Baeppler who has spent long hours helping me refine the text and to Mark Tillotson for his creative and technical help in formatting the book. It might have remained simply a good idea without the enthusiasm and belief of the current and former commissioning editors at Butterworth-Heinemann, Mary Seager and Susan Devlin, who have conjured up a 'fresh breeze' during periods when both I and the book have been in the doldrums.

Part

1

Meaning and behaviour

Introduction

Over the latter decades of the last century a quiet revolution has been taking place in mental health care as humanistic ideas have gradually permeated and embedded themselves in the practice, education and management. It is the premise of this section of the book that a humanistic philosophy now provides the most relevant theoretical foundation on which to build the practice of mental health nursing. I use the term philosophy both to reflect the origins of humanistic ideas, many of which have their roots in existent-ialism, and to reflect the core themes of this book which are concerned with the values that underpin professional helping.

In Chapter 1, the humanistic lens is applied to the experience of disabling distress which, it is argued, can only be understood from the perspective of the individual seeking help. It takes a holistic view, seeing distress behaviour as an outcome of disharmony in the biological, psycho-social and spiritual dimensions of human experience.

Well-being depends not just on inner harmony but also on being 'in communion' with the social context in which we live out our lives. Chapter 2 considers the social and cultural context of distress and makes a case for an anti-oppressive approach to mental health care in which social disadvantage and oppression are given the attention they deserve.

The theme of Chapter 3 is working creatively with people in crisis. Distress can at times be so overwhelming that a person's mental and social functioning becomes seriously disturbed. Currently a lot of endeavour is going into developing crisis services in which crisis is perceived not as a sign of failure on the part of the service user or the practitioners, but as a learning opportunity. A crisis is seen not as another breakdown, but as another opportunity for a breakthrough.

Chapter 4 outlines a holistic, person-centred, approach to assessment. It steers a course away from the pseudo-science of assessment tools and dia-gnostic interviews that attempt to fit the experience of individuals into pathologized conceptions of distress. It argues instead for an empathic dialogue in which the experience of the client is made known and its meaning in the context of their lives understood.

In Chapter 5, the recovery process comes into focus. Recovery can be seen as a continuing journey towards a higher level of well-being and in that sense it is a journey we all share. Psychiatry is not very good at sowing seeds of hope. A culture of maintenance, rather than recovery, dominates the psychiatric stage, in which the troubled individual is cast as a prisoner of their biology and destined to live a life circumscribed by their continuing vulnerability. The missing ingredient here is realistic hopefulness. Hope for a less anguished way of being in the world. Hope for an ordinary life. Mental health professionals need to be able to hold hope for those seeking care and become companions on their journeys of recovery.

Chapter 6 is an exploration of a philosophy of care based on humanistic principles. Compassionate care is the art of being rather than doing. It is about being with people in a way which is respectful, empathic and enabling, which nourishes the growth of the troubled individual towards becoming a fully functioning person who has the resourcefulness to manage the problems and opportunities of living.

The nature of human distress

The humanistic, person-centred approach to understanding and helping people who are deeply distressed is rooted in the phenomenological tradition of Western philosophy. The phenomenological view of man does not try to impose any theoretical construct on that experience, but seeks to make sense of distressed and disturbed behaviour principally through an understanding of a person's subjective world. In so doing it unshackles differentness from pathology. Experiencing the world or oneself in unusual ways may be problematic and disturbing for the individual and others, but it is not a phenomenon that is outside the range of 'normal' human experience. As Chadwick (1996) argues, the assumption of a discontinuity between ordinary experience and psychotic experience is imaginary. Many people have strongly held unusual beliefs, which have many of the characteristics of beliefs that, in a psychiatric context, would be considered delusional and symptomatic of psychosis. But, however unusual an individual's beliefs might be about himself and his world, they can usually be understood in relation to his life experience. Similarly, voice hearing may be a cause of distress and problematic behaviour, but many people who are not considered psychotic experience voices. Romme and Escher (1993), in their seminal work on voice hearing, make the case that the nature and content of voices always has meaning in the context of the person's life.

Perhaps, as Rogers (1978a) suggests, there is not one reality but multiple realities experienced at both a cultural and individual level.

> The only reality I can know for certain is the world as I perceive and experience it at this moment. The only reality you can know for certain is the world as you perceive and experience it at this moment. The only certainty is that they are not the same (p. 424).

Rogers argues that, rather than try to change a person's reality, the task of helping is to respect and understand his view of himself in the world. If we can relate to people in respectful, authentic and empathic ways, the most troubled and alienated person will be literally brought to his senses. That is, he will become more in touch with his true being and become more fully, rather than selectively, aware of the physical and interpersonal world in which he lives. Reality is largely relational with us testing out the validity of our perceptions and experience in the social matrix of our everyday lives. Though differing fundamentally from Rogers' approach, cognitive behavioural ways of working with unusual beliefs that are problematic and distressing to the individual are, in essence, strategic ways of reality testing. Central to this process is establishing that what the client experiences is a belief and not objective reality.

The humanistic view of man is basically optimistic, holding that, given favourable conditions for development, we move towards becoming fully functioning people who behave in socially constructive ways. Rogers characterized the fully functioning person as someone open to the experience of themselves, others and the world. If we can be sufficiently open to experience and not subject it to defensive distortion, we are able to engage more freely and creatively in the process of living. Rogers argues that the more open to experience we are, the more we are able to trust our 'felt sense', our emotional intelligence and intuition, in concert with cognitive evaluation, to inform our choices and decisions. This more holistic way of being leads to wise action. The journey towards becoming more fully ourselves, what Abraham Maslow called self-actualization, lies at the heart of humanistic and existential thinking about psychological well-being and disturbance. If we become alienated from our true selves and live our lives in an inauthentic way, we will find it difficult to know what we truly think or feel, or to express our needs and so act in constructive ways when faced with the challenges of living. We will then be at risk of becoming overwhelmed by accumulating distress.

People who have never achieved this strong sense of their own identity and reality are particularly vulnerable to the vicissitudes and adversities of everyday life. Escaping into madness can sometimes seem preferable to the continuing struggle. Such crisis-prone individuals may frequently spiral down into a state of despair, confusion and chaos. This does not mean that people with this high level of vulnerability necessarily require a sheltered existence and medication that blurs their reality. Disturbance and crisis from a humanistic and existential framework are seen as experiential learning opportunities from which a stronger sense of self and reality can develop.

The quest for selfhood begins in infancy and childhood, during which time our emergent sense of self is particularly vulnerable to approval and validation by the significant care givers in our lives. In unfavourable circumstances, the care we receive may be conditional on our being and behaving in certain ways, which limits the expression of our unfolding self. In these circumstances, our self-concept is created out of the internalized conditions of worth imposed on us by others, rather than by the prompting of our true self. The internalized beliefs and values of others may be difficult to live up to. We will often fall short of those standards and, as a consequence, develop a deeply negative sense of self which, once established, will produce behaviour that reflects and confirms our negative self-evaluation. Similarly, traumatic experiences of loss or abuse that deprive us of secure, nurturing relationships can dislocate us from what we have the potential to be. Individuals who come to see themselves as inadequate are likely to live their life in restricted ways and depend on others for solutions to the challenges of everyday living. The belief that 'I can't' rather than the belief that 'I can' becomes the credo by which such individuals live their lives. People with deeply negative self-concepts do not have that inner core of self-worth that comes from the experience of having one's emergent self prized and nurtured during early development. Their self-esteem will be low and externally regulated, vulnerable to the rejections, disappointments and failures that are part of human experience.

Most of us accumulate some distress as we grow up and grow older. This distress is held in the body-mind and we acquire various strategies to defend ourselves against it in an attempt to prevent it surfacing into awareness and overwhelming us. Those who carry high levels of distress are likely to lead a life restricted by defensive behaviour. They live on the edge of their distress and are at risk of being emotionally overwhelmed by the problems of living (Figure 1.1). Archaic distress is always likely to be re-activated by stressful events in the here and now, particularly those that in some way mirror earlier experiences. People who are highly vulnerable to this psycho-social overwhelm may adopt extreme strategies in order to try to cope. They may shut down or harm themselves in an attempt to deal with overwhelming feelings of despair, helplessness, anger, guilt or self-loathing. They may begin to hear voices or develop unusual beliefs as a way of coping with their inner distress or become so withdrawn and reclusive that they are difficult to reach. It is this 'distress behaviour' that is often pathologized, explained as psychiatric disorder and suppressed by powerful neuroleptic drugs.

So universal is the experience of archaic distress that it is frequently represented in folk tales by the image of the dragon's cave. This is portrayed as a fearful place, which the hero enters, usually after a perilous journey, to defeat the dragon and discover the treasure that the dragon guards. It involves facing what is difficult to face, discovering the treasure within

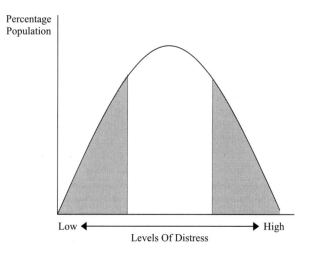

Figure 1.1 Levels of distress in the general population. Epidemiological studies estimate that the prevalence of high levels of distress likely to express itself in mental health problems is between 260 and 315 people per 1000 of the population annually. Approximately 24 people per 1000 are likely to become mental health service users annually (Goldberg and Huxley, 1992)

and emerging with a stronger sense of self, a more positive self-evaluation and less reliance on defensive behaviour. This heroic journey can be seen as a metaphor for therapeutic endeavour, often undertaken with help and companionship. I do not mean to suggest by this some 'revelatory, cathartic, couch experience', more a continuing journey of self-discovery that is part of a living-learning experience.

Being authentic, being true to oneself, is not about living without regard for others – a cult of individualism. In fact the opposite is true. The more we are in touch with and express who we are, the more empathic and connected we are with others. Without empathy there could be no intimacy or cohesiveness in social relationships. Neither is authenticity a way of being that disregards constraints. The reality of human existence is that the freedom to be oneself is inevitably constrained by the social systems and political realities that impact on our lived experience.

While the powerful influence of inheritance, our psychological environment and social circumstances on our way of being is not denied, the perspective of humanistic philosophy is not to see people as prisoners of their biology or their past or present circumstances. There is a belief in the essential freedom and responsibility of human beings to recreate themselves and their lives. If we are in the process of becoming fully functioning people, we are in touch with our personal power and self-agency. We can transcend adversity and adjust to changing circumstances. Being authentic allows us to face reality and not distort it or deny it in order to protect our false and fragile self-concept. The basis of much disabling distress and disturbance has its origins in this self-deception. For example, the failure to own certain emotions may mean that they are denied or projected on to others, with the consequence that we relate to others in an inauthentic way and have a distorted view of reality.

This way of conceptualizing growth as a realization of the attributes that define us as individuals and human beings, who are nourished and influenced by family experience and culture and by the choices we make about our way of being in the world, is but one view. It is a view challenged by some who see the idea of self as highly individualized and autonomous as an ethnocentric Western concept (Holdstock, 1993). In many non-Western cultures, the self is constituted much more by the social context, within which integration and harmony are valued. Fernando (1995) argues that integration, balance and harmony within oneself and within the family and community are important aspects of what may be considered mental health in traditional non-Western cultures while, in the West, self-sufficiency, autonomy, the enhancement of self and self-esteem are important criteria. Westernized constructs of mental health and psychological distress and disturbance that are universally applied in a multiethnic society are untenable. Knowledge of what is normal and what is pathological is shaped by cultural definitions of personhood, social identities and role expectation (Ahmed and Webb Johnson, 1995). Any psychiatric assessment must take into account a person's culturally determined beliefs about the cause of their distress and what *they* think would be acceptable and helpful interventions in restoring their well-being. For some clients, spiritual care from leaders of their faith community may be seen as more relevant than a pharmacological or psychotherapeutic intervention.

Another challenge to the concept of separation and individuation has come from feminist writers who argue that this is more a male conceptualization than female. Women, it is argued, do not set themselves so sharply apart. The boundaried self is more permeable and their way of being in the world more relational than for men. For women, connection and embeddedness within social groups is of vital importance for the emergence of identity. The 'me' is derived from 'we' (Josselyn, 1987). Unlike males, who grow up in a culture that stresses self-assertion, mastery, individual distinction and separation, women are raised in a culture that emphasizes communion. Skills and successes in relatedness become the keystones of identity.

Ian's story *(Theme: vulnerability to psycho-social overwhelm and disabling distress)*

I've been seeing psychiatrists for the last 10 years for schizophrenia, since I was 18. I'm better than I was. I used to feel drugged up, like my body didn't belong to me. Now I have quite a low dose of my medication by injection and take extra tablets if I feel I need it. What stresses me most is feeling bored and lonely. My life feels empty a lot of the time. It's then that my voices become worse and bother me more. I hear several voices, usually bad mouthing me, calling me a 'waste of space' or 'a loser'. Sometimes I feel depressed about my life and think about ending it; I did stab myself in the chest once. Some people seem to get over schizophrenia but for me it's always there; that's what frightens me, this feeling that it's who I am. Often it's difficult to make sense of things. Little things can trouble me for ages. I saw some girls laughing in town the other day, one of them was on her mobile phone and I thought why am I suffering and they're laughing. Then I began to think I was a scapegoat, carrying all the blame for other people. I got the feeling I had been banished and that everyone wanted me gone.

What I need is a girlfriend and a job. But that's difficult. I haven't got much confidence and I worry about how people will react when they know I've been in a mental hospital and I'm on medication. It's hard to get a foothold in the world when you've been ill. I remember when I came out of hospital the second time, I felt utterly helpless, I just couldn't cope and went high. I started thinking I was on TV, a star in a soap and that cameras were filming me. I miss that feeling of being high even though I know I had some crazy ideas. It was a bit like taking a holiday in an exotic place.

It would be easy to become a full-time patient, mix with other service users, go to the resource centre or join one of the work projects, but I want an ordinary life. I did three months' voluntary conservation work three summers ago and I was hoping to do a part-time environmental studies course but I became unwell again just before the term started. Now I'm not sure I could cope with it.

I think my schizophrenia started when I was a child. My father left when I was seven. I used to see him at weekends, then he got married again and stopped coming. I wasn't important enough to him I suppose. Then my mother's new partner started to knock her about, he couldn't stand to have me around so I went and lived with my Grandma for about a year till my mother left him. I hated school. I was an outsider even then and was bullied from when I was about nine until I was thirteen. The teachers used to say I was vacant and I was. I went a long way away, deep inside and lost myself.

Francine's story *(Theme: vulnerability to psycho-social overwhelm and disabling distress)*
I'm 53 now and have suffered from anxiety and depression for the past 11 years. I find it difficult being on my own and get panicky. I don't really know why I should so feel so helpless and worried. I know it frustrates my husband that I rely on him so much. Going out is difficult as I find it hard to talk to people. I worry that everyone will know I've been in hospital and that they will be thinking I'm a loathsome person for not getting over this and looking after my family properly. I've had so much help from everyone – doctors, nurses, my psychologist, I'm sure they are all getting fed up with me. When I'm very depressed, I get frightening thoughts that seem very real at the time, that I've done something terrible and that it's in all the newspapers. At times in the past I've been so overwhelmed with worry and just wanted it to stop that I've tried to kill myself.

My life is quite empty really. I should have gone back to work after Julian (son) left school but I never felt confident enough or skilled enough and I didn't think they would want me. Also I wanted another baby but it didn't happen. When I look back on my life I've always had people to look after, now there's no one. My mother suffered from multiple sclerosis. My older sister and I used to look after her when she became very disabled. Then she died. I remember the house feeling very empty. My dad was good to us but he was not someone you could easily confide in or go to if you were upset. He became a strict Methodist after my mother's death and we were encouraged to look to God for comfort and guidance. I think I grew up feeling that I had to be good and that meant being nice and not making a fuss about anything. I remember being terrified by the idea that God could look into my heart and discover what a despicable child I was.

I'm not sure what's going to happen to me, but I am feeling a bit more hopeful. It's about 18 months since I last had to go into hospital. I'm still taking regular medication, although it hasn't really helped me much. I see my community nurse once a week and we work on building up coping strategies and I also have a support worker. If I get very low now I can check myself into The Moorings (a woman's respite and recovery house). I have experienced a lot of love and care there. I remember the first time I was there one of the women sat up half the night just holding me. It was the first time I can remember feeling safe.

Social and cultural issues in the experience of distress

2

The problems faced by long-term service users are often more social than psychiatric. The difficulties they face have less to do with a continuing vulnerability to disabling distress and more to do with the experience of being marginalized and stigmatized. Social exclusion results not just from prejudicial attitudes towards people with mental health problems, but is also the result of impoverishment. The emphasis on growth and enterprise in the UK has resulted in a growing underclass, of which those with enduring mental illness are a proportionately large number, who find themselves in persistent poverty and separated from the rest of us (Barham and Hayward, 1995). Hopton (1997) argues strongly for mental health nursing to develop an anti-oppressive approach to practice, an approach emphasizing the social, cultural and political environment as the primary source of clients' distress.

Surveys of public attitudes towards mental health care resources being located in the community often reveal high levels of opposition (Repper *et al.*, 1997). This opposition can take the form of letters of protest, protest meetings, the circulation of offensive leaflets, graffiti and slogans painted on walls and hostility towards service providers and users. Such attitudes are mostly based on misunderstanding and ignorance. Fears arise from the widely held perception that people with severe mental health problems are often 'out of control' or 'unpredictable' and may pose a threat. The way severe mental distress is portrayed by the media creates images of danger-ousness in the minds of the public. Such tabloid images can also be dam-aging to the morale and self-concept of people who have been diagnosed as having schizophrenia, forcing them into a reclusive life style (Philo, 1997).

As Barham and Hayward suggest, stigma such as this can create a scenario where,

> 'the ex-mental patient finds himself nominally a citizen alongside others, but by virtue of a history of mental illness, continued vulnerability and disability, bar-riers to participation in social life, and the uncertain reception often accorded to them, they find themselves as separated and isolated as if they were hidden away in the asylum' (p. 144).

In practice the outcome is not always so gloomy. Repper *et al.* (1997) observe that mental health users themselves are the best ambassadors for community-based services. Once living and working in a neighbourhood and using the same community facilities as everyone else, they are accepted – neither causing problems nor attracting hostility from the local residents.

Many users of mental health services are engaged in a daily struggle with poverty. Poverty reduces choices and opportunities. It can mean insufficient food, inadequate clothing, poor quality housing, a bleak non-sustaining living space, and restricted social and leisure opportunities. Poverty, as much as disability, separates people from the mainstream of community life. To feel trapped in an impoverished life is a major cause of distress. If you take any neighbourhood with a high rate of premature death and serious physical illness, then it is likely that the neighbourhood will be a poor one and that it will also show a high rate of suicide, depression, anxiety states and schizophrenia (Gomm, 1996).

Many people who use the mental health services see overcoming the impoverishment of their lives as the factor that would lead to the most significant improvement to their mental health. As Brandon (1991) argues, poverty and powerlessness are the most important symptoms of mental illness. Yet this important social dimension is often neglected and not addressed in practice by mental health practitioners. Davis and Wainwright (1996) suggest that behind this neglect is often the belief that impoverishment is, at least in part, self-inflicted, the result of the fecklessness of service users. The prevalence of judgemental attitudes is one reason why service users do not always seek help from statutory services to negotiate the benefit system and deal with debt. Instead, they seek support from welfare rights advisers and independent advocates where they are available. There is a need for mental health professionals and service providers to become more aware of the impact of poverty and committed to anti-poverty action in their practice and provision.

A charter for poverty awareness and anti-poverty action

- Recognize the social, psychological, physical impact of poverty on service users.
- Recognize the stigma and discrimination faced by service user claimants.
- Gain sufficient knowledge of welfare rights and entitlement to provide advice and support to service users in making claims that maximize their income.
- Work with service users in an empowering enabling way in managing benefits and dealing with debts.
- Recognize the experience and 'expertise' of some service users in relation to welfare rights and benefits. Involve them in staff training events.
- Support the training and development of welfare rights advisers and debt counsellors within the user movement.
- Provide good quality affordable housing.
- Create opportunities for work and training, including collective work, that will combat poverty.

(Adapted from Davis and Wainwright, 1996)

Work is important in all our lives and not simply for the income it provides. It gives us a valued social role and contributes to our sense of identity. The status and role work provides are critical to someone who only has the devalued identity of 'mental patient' (Perkins and Repper, 1996). Work provides us with a source of satisfaction and achievement and supports our self-esteem. It also creates opportunities for social relationships, support and friendship. It is hardly surprising then that unemployment significantly affects mental health or that socially valued, meaningful employment can make a significant difference to the well-being of people with long-term mental health problems. The desire to be gainfully employed is an expressed need of most long-term service users, the majority of whom are unemployed. Given that entry into open employment is often difficult, there is a need for more community-based work projects providing meaningful, socially valued occupations such as those described by Nehring *et al.* (1993). Such projects are outward looking, involving project workers within the wider community. They create an empowering and supportive context in which people can increase their income, gain skills and confidence and have a real say in the development and management of the project. For some, such initiatives provide a pathway back into open employment. Despite the need for such projects, we should not be deflected from the aim of gaining access to open employment for people with disabilities. Perkins and Repper argue that it is the work setting that has to change in order to accommodate people with mental health disabilities and promote social inclusiveness. While some employers have adapted their work environments and practices to meet the needs of people with physical disabilities and learning disabilities, few have been flexible enough to accommodate people with psychosocial disabilities.

Yet there are innovative examples, such as transitional employment schemes organized by the clubhouse movement. The Health Service on the other hand, one of the biggest employers in the UK, has been slow to lead the way in offering employment to service users in clinical posts and support services, despite the success of such schemes in America (Sherman and Porter, 1991).

A high priority for service users is access to decent housing, somewhere to feel at home and secure. People who do not have accommodation when they could be discharged continue to block acute hospital beds and often end up in inappropriate bed and breakfast accommodation or hostels for the homeless. Studies of the homeless population of the UK suggest the proportion with mental illness is between 30 and 40%, of whom many will suffer from schizophrenia (Mental Health Foundation, 1997). Some will have additional problems, such as multiple substance abuse. Homelessness exacerbates mental and physical health problems and it can be difficult for mental health practitioners to stay in contact with clients. One of the key issues in the housing provision for vulnerable people is that it should be available with care and support. Tenancies can often break down and result in homelessness if people do not receive the support they need. Tenancies break down because of rent arrears, failure to care appropriately for the accommodation or because of problems with the neighbours. There is a clear need for more housing to be made available to people with long-term mental health problems ranging from 24-hour-staffed accommodation to supported self-contained flats. But, if social inclusiveness is to become a reality, it is important the housing provision moves away from specialist accommodation towards providing people with enough support to maintain a place of their own in the open housing market.

What are the implications of all this for the helping relationship? It is clearly important to acknowledge the impact on psychological well-being of stigma, discrimination, social impoverishment and disadvantage. In reality the recognition of this is often only cursory. The mental health services are dominated by models that locate dysfunction within the individual that must be put right by therapy, rather than within a dysfunctional society that seems to have lost its capacity to care and has largely abdicated that moral responsibility to professional carers. Smails (1998) in a powerful argument on the limits of therapy takes the view that we cling to a 'therapeutic illusion', that a history of, for example, abuse and social deprivation which expresses itself in distress and disturbance can be wiped away. At best therapy is palliative. What is needed is a political and ethical current that shifts society towards a more caring and egalitarian way of being.

Davidson (1998), drawing on Smails' work, suggests that the role of the nurse is to try to understand and demystify the problems the client faces and to see that these are not the product of pathological processes, but an understandable way of being and surviving, given their history and experience. A normalizing stance such as this is difficult to hold on to. First, a reductionist medical view of the problem is often easier both for the client and the nurse, rather than attempting to identify and confront the deprivation and abuse that has been the client's experience. Facing the hurt perpetrated by others, the hurt done to others, and identifying injustice and oppression does not magically cure the client, but places distress in its rightful context and does not seek to obscure it with diagnostic labels and pathologizing processes.

Davidson argues that, in addition to demystifying the client's problems, the role of the nurse is to be a comforting, nurturing, encouraging presence. Drawing on his own experience of working with people with complex problems of living, he argues that,

> 'if we can just be with someone no matter what state they are in, without needing to act on them or change them, yet be vibrantly alive to their humanity, then clients do eventually feel sufficiently safe and courageous to tackle aspects of their life which are amenable to development' (p. 63).

Creating this healing ground in the interface between people is more about ways of being in relationship with people in care than what we do. This clearly has implications for the professional education of mental health nurses where the 'knowledgeable doer' is valued more than learning to be in a therapeutic alliance with clients.

Transcultural issues

Does similarity of age, cultural and social background, the same gender and sexual orientation make any difference to the sense of connection and the ability of the helper to work in culturally sensitive ways? Dupont-Joshua (1996) argues that it is important not to deny differentness in helping relationships, particularly where there is an ethnicity or gender difference. It can often seem safer to hide behind statements such as, 'It makes no difference to me what a person's ethnic background is', or, 'I treat all my clients the same'. But to do so is to deny what we represent on a symbolic level to the client and lose an opportunity to work with some of the issues that are part of the client's wider social experience that has contributed to their distress. To do so also adds to a client's sense of 'invisibility' in that their essential being is not 'seen' and respected. We cannot be neutral. We bring to the helping relationship consciously or unconsciously our racist attitudes. A starting point is openly to acknowledge this: 'I don't know too much about your culture of origin, I will be interested to hear about your experience of it as we talk'; 'I may at times say things which seem culturally insensitive or uninformed and if I do, I hope you will point that out to me'; 'Because of our different ethnic backgrounds, there are bound to be issues for both of us to consider in our work together, but they could be more of a help than a hindrance'; ' I'm wondering how you feel about being referred to me, a white person with little experience of your culture?' References to helping relationships in the literature refer mostly to white helpers and black (and other ethnic minority) clients, but is important to recognize that issues can arise which can impede the development and therapeutic helpfulness of the relationship when the position is reversed. Dupont-Joshua refers to the tendency of some white clients to 'mythologize' black mental health workers, bringing archaic fears and fantasies to the surface. However, while there is clearly a need for all nurses to be conscious of their own racist and oppressive attitudes and to seek to relate to people from ethnic minorities in sensitive, informed ways, it is also important not to lose an awareness of commonalities. It is our shared humanness that connects us.

Policy documents on ethnicity and mental health nursing (MIND, 1993; Royal College of Nursing, 1996) recommend a recruitment policy that reflects the ethnicity structure of the local populations. They also point to a need for better information about services; access to professional interpreters; the availability of advocacy from a person of the same cultural background and a more influential role for the user/survivor movement. While the user/survivor movement in the UK includes many members from the ethnic minorities, it has been criticized for having a white Western perspective that inadequately represents the experience of black users (Sassoon and Lindow 1995). A predominantly white user group can be an oppressive context for a black survivor to articulate their experience of racism within the mental health system and in society at large. Although still far too few, there is a growing number of innovative and black and Asian user projects which provide an empowering social context in which support and advocacy can be provided to users and consultancy offered to service providers on the development and effectiveness of services to ethnic minority groups. An excellent example is KUSH in the London Borough of Hackney who provide housing, a crisis sanctuary and an outreach crisis service to the local African and Caribbean communities (Mental Health Foundation, 1997).

The White City Project, now called the Centre for Women's Emotional Well Being, is another example of how innovation in community mental health care can be empowering to socially disadvantaged groups and lead to the development of an autonomous service that challenges the doctrine that professionals as opposed to lay helpers know what is best (Holland, 1995). The project has its roots firmly in a multicultural, working-class community and has as a theoretical base social action psychotherapy, a model that confronts both psychological distress and social oppression. This process of empowerment involves stepping out of the passive patient/victim role, finding meaning for present distress in past oppression, engaging support groups in which the shared social history of participants emerges. Freed from the constraints of the past, social action to meet the needs of the present becomes a possibility.

Although many social groups in our society have experienced discrimination and oppression within the psychiatric system, it is particularly so for Afro-Caribbean, Asian and other minority ethnic groups. Racism is, of course, not confined to the mental health services, but permeates all social institutions – education, criminal justice system, local authority services, social services. It seems only belatedly, following public enquiries such as the shaming Stephen Lawrence enquiry, that the existence of institutional racism at the core of our institutions is being acknowledged and confronted. The reality of racism within the mental health services has been highlighted by studies over the past 20 years which show significant cultural variations in the experience of psychiatric services between white British and people from ethnic minority groups.

Institutional racism in mental health services

Black people are more likely than white:
- To be diagnosed as suffering from schizophrenia or another form of psychosis.
- To be detained in a locked ward or secure psychiatric unit.
- To be detained in hospital under Sections 2, 3 and 4 of the Mental Health Act 1983.
- To be removed to a place of safety by the police under Section 136.
- To be given higher doses of medication.
- To experience unmet needs.

They are less likely:
- To be referred for psychotherapy or counselling.
- To receive an appropriate assessment and intervention at an early stage.

(Source: Department of Health and Home Office, 1992)

The dominant discourse on severe distress in our culture is an ethnocentric Western view, which conceptualizes it as a dysfunctional state located within the individual. So dominant is this illness hypothesis that it has achieved the status of a truth and provides the authoritative base for professional, expert-led care. While the conception of distress as illness to be treated by health care professionals may be relevant and acceptable to many people seeking help, it is often inappropriate to people whose social experience and beliefs are rooted in non-Western cultures. Furthermore, racial stereotyping, cultural insensitivity and oppressive practices that are often the experience of black and other ethnic minority users of the psychiatric system, increase the reluctance of people to access services. The idea that recovery of well-being requires the intervention of psychiatrists, psychologists and nurses is not a belief that is readily accepted by all cultures, where ideas of what constitutes the conditions for healing and recovery might have a different emphasis. If depression is experienced more as oppression, then it is not treatment that is required, but social action. If unusual thoughts or voice hearing relate to the spiritual realm of a person's life, then it is maybe the leader of their faith community who should be consulted. If the problem is perceived as a loss of harmony, either in a person's inner or outer world, then it may be that consulting a healer, complementary therapist or talking with a trusted elder would be a more acceptable course of action. For some, the manifestation of distress may be seen as a problem requiring family care, rather than the intrusive intervention of some outside agency. But it is a mistake to think that the cultural identity of a client necessarily determines their conception of the problem and what needs to be done about it. Fernando (1995) argues that culture is not a fixed entity, but an 'emergent' process that is influenced by the social and family context as much as by tradition. To make assumptions about an individual's mental health needs simply by reference to their cultural group leads to stereotyping, for example, that 'British Asians have close supportive extended families by comparison with British whites'. There is also a tendency to classify people whose origins are geographically similar into one group, for example South-East Asians, ignoring the rich diversity of beliefs and traditions that exist in cultures rooted in that part of the world. Training in relation to ethnicity, as with gender, often misses the essential point that the main focus needs to be internal, raising awareness of personal rather than external attitudes, and focusing on increasing factual knowledge of a particular culture. Taking a more fluid view of culture frees us from relying too much on having detailed knowledge of a cultural group in order to be sensitive in assessing needs and allows us to draw much more on the unique experience of the individual or family.

Conditions for healing. A comparison of Eastern and Western beliefs

Eastern	Western
Acceptance	Regaining autonomy and control
Regain harmony and integration	Problem solving
Holistic awareness	Cognitive understanding
Contemplation/prayer	Body–mind separation
Unity of body–mind–spirit	Recovery of self
Ethical way of being	Recovery of self-esteem
Self-help through family/ community 'healers'	Expert-dependent help through psychiatric system

(Adapted from Fernando, 1995)

Self-enquiry Box

To split beliefs about healing into an Eastern and Western tradition does not accurately reflect reality. It is seldom so clear cut in a multi-ethnic society such as Britain. Many individuals whose origins are in white Western culture have beliefs around healing that would fit more comfortably with an Eastern approach.

Explore your own beliefs about healing:
- *What stories were you told about illness and healing as you were growing up? What effect did they have on you?*
- *Who was the 'healer' in your family as you were growing up?*
- *When you think of illness, which words and images come to mind?*
- *When you think of healing, which words and images come to mind?*
- *How have you healed yourself at times when you've been physically unwell?*
- *How have you healed yourself at times when you've experienced psychological hurt?*
- *Do you recognize messages in your body/mind symptoms?*
- *Who have been the healers in your experiences of physical ill health?*
- *Who have been the healers when you have experienced psychological distress?*
- *What words and images come to mind when you think of a place of healing?*

Self-enquiry Box

An anti-oppressive approach to mental health nursing

- *Mental health nurses should recognize that a person's mental distress is at least in part the product of his or her social, political and cultural environment.*
- *Nursing assessments should be orientated towards helping clients reflect on their social, political and cultural experience (including the psychiatric system) so as to identify aspects of the environment that are oppressive and distressing.*
- *Nursing interventions should be orientated towards helping clients make conscious choices about whether they wish to engage in social action or some other course of action in response to the cause of their distress.*
- *Mental health nurses should relate to clients in a way that enables them to discover their own power, feel more in control of their lives and strengthens their self-esteem.*

(Source: Hopton, 1997, p. 878)

Consider what changes you would need to make to your practice in order to work with people in an anti-oppressive way, more completely and more of the time. Try to be specific.

Gender issues: the experience of women

An area of concern in relation to anti-oppressive practice is the experience of women users of the mental health services. A growing body of literature over the past two decades has drawn attention to the patriarchal nature of large parts of the mental health service (Showalter, 1987; Usser, 1991). The charge is that mental health professionals have consistently failed to respond to, and in some cases have reinforced, the experience of social inequality, disempowerment and abuse that is, for many women, a social reality and a major factor in their distressed and disturbed behaviour. Additionally, recent reports (Sainsbury Centre, 1998b) have drawn attention to the dissatisfaction of many women with acute inpatient services, which often do not provide them with the privacy, sense of safety and freedom from sexual harassment, that should be fundamental elements in a caring environment.

Contact with the mental health services often comes about as the result of sexual, physical or emotional abuse, experienced both as children and as adults. There is strong evidence that this is a major factor contributing to women's mental health problems, including the diagnosis of severe mental illness (Goodman *et al.*, 1993; Polusny and Follette, 1995). Given the high incidence of an experience of abuse among female users, it is essential that mental health workers have the sensitivity and awareness to address this as a possibility in their conversations with clients. Not to do so is to replicate the experience of not being heard and helped and to reinforce the sense of blame, shame and guilt common in the histories of abused women. There clearly needs to be not just a greater awareness of abuse, but a pool of skilled help available both within and outside the mental health services.

Social inequalities, which are more frequently experienced by women, also correlate with psychological distress and referral to the mental health services. Recent reports (Department of Health, 1994) have highlighted the need for mental health workers to recognize, in their work with clients, the significance of social issues and intervene in ways that seek to ameliorate these as causes of distress. The experience of women of professional carers is still too often of not being listened to, of routinized treatment, of high doses of psychotrophic drugs and frequent admissions to inpatient units (Williams and Watson, 1996). Although the use of ECT is declining in the UK, approximately 1300 are still administered each week, of which 68% are to women. Rowe (1996) suggests that recurrent depression in women is more likely to be seen as an internal event, unrelated to the cultural and social circumstances, to be treated by physical means.

The mental health consequences of the social and cultural realities of women

- Marriage is more likely to be beneficial to the psychological well-being of men and detrimental to the well-being of women.
- Childbirth is linked with depression for a significant number of women.
- Caring for children and dependent relatives carries a high emotional cost when associated with isolation, low social value and lack of resources.
- The link between poverty and a higher incidence of psychological ill health is well documented. Poverty among women is strongly asso-

ciated with being a single parent, being divorced, being old and being a member of an ethnic minority group.
- Domestic violence is estimated to occur in 1 in 4 households in the UK, largely perpetrated by men towards women. Links between domestic violence and mental health difficulties are now well established.
- 1 in 4 women have been victims of rape or sexual assault. Victimization is a powerful predictor of mental health problems.
- It is estimated that between 1 in 3 and 1 in 10 girls are sexually abused in childhood, an experience that can have a profound effect on mental health.
- Women's feelings, thoughts and behaviours are more likely to be defined as madness than men's.

(Source: Williams and Watson, 1996)

What is crucial is that the education of mental health workers should provide an opportunity to develop a critical awareness of the experience, needs and resourcefulness of women seeking help. This learning can come from various sources: listening more to women users; by women's groups being involved in training mental health workers; from women-centred mental health projects; and from the growing body of literature. An increased awareness can also be derived from our own experience of oppression and entrapment.

Self-enquiry Box

Make a list of statements about yourself and your life beginning with the phrase I must ....

Put this list of statements out of sight and complete a second list beginning with the phrase I choose ....

Now compare the two lists. Consider the extent to which your way of being is a self-determined choice and how much is an expression of the internalized expectations from your family and the wider culture.

Self-enquiry Box

The following exercise can be a useful way of identifying unacknowledged resentments and uncovering the unexpressed appreciations you feel in relation to significant people in your life and the various roles you play. The exercise may enable you to articulate these feelings more assertively.

Make a list of all the things that you resent:
About the way you are treated as a man/as a woman.
About the way you are treated as a gay man/lesbian.
About the way you are treated by your parents/ your partner/ your children.
About the way you are treated as an employee.
About the way you are treated as a citizen.

When you have completed one of the above categories, think about the 'demands' that underlie the resentments and capture them as written

statements. Try to be as clear and direct as you can as in the example below.
Resentment 'I resent the way you treat me like a child'.
Demand 'I want you to respect my decisions and choices'.
Now using the same category list all of the things that you appreciate.
Reflect on your lists and consider how you might use what you have learnt as a basis for personal or social action.

Self-enquiry Box

The drama triangle is a powerful way of analysing a form of role-playing that commonly occurs both in social and professional relationships. These are inauthentic roles based on old script strategies that have their origins in the past, rather than the here and now. Stewart and Joines (1987) describe a persecutor as someone who puts down other people and be-littles them. The persecutor views others as being 'one down' and 'not OK'. A rescuer also sees others as 'not OK' and 'one down' but responds by offering or imposing help from a 'one up' position. The rescuer's belief is that they have to help because others are not able to cope. The victim sees himself as 'not OK' and in the 'one down' position. Victims will search out a persecutor who will put them down, confirming their view of themselves. Other victims will search for a rescuer to confirm their view that they can't cope on their own. All three roles involve a 'discount'. The persecutor discounts others value, dignity and well-being. The rescuer discounts others' ability to think for themselves and use their own initiative. The victim discounts him- or herself; seeing themselves as deserving denigra-tion or needing help in order to cope and survive. Although people may seem stuck in a particular role, they are also likely to switch to another role in playing out their scripts. A victim may become a persecutor, a rescuer may become a victim.

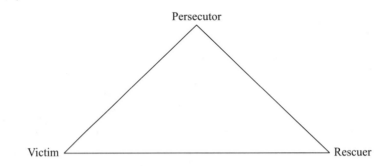

Take a few minutes to brainstorm all the words you associate with the three roles.

Consider what the differences are between an authentic rescuer and an inauthentic one. Can you make the same distinction for victims?

Reflect on your own experience of occupying these roles, through being 'recruited' into one, having one imposed on you, or through acting out your own script in your personal and professional life.

Gender issues: the experience of men

Over the past few decades much of the debate on gender has rightly addressed the experience of women. More recently, the well-being of men and the position of men in society has come into focus. Tremendous changes have taken place in the lives of men over the latter half of this century. The declining industrial base and the disappearance of traditional labour inten- sive industries has robbed men of the occupational roles from which they once drew their sense of identity. In the process the 'lessons in masculinity' that were absorbed from the work culture are no longer available. The 'new man' who began to emerge in the liberal culture of the 1960s, which created a social climate in which men could develop their feminine side, has left men feeling incomplete. While there is satisfaction for many men in being able to develop and express a more sensitive, caring, feeling side, it has been at the expense of the positive energy of masculine aggression. There needs to be a balance; to be defined by qualities most often associated with femininity can be threatening to most men. Male aggression and sexuality have been de- monized in our culture, where they have become linked with wife beating, child abuse and criminality. It is an image that makes it difficult to accept and integrate positive masculine energy, and allow it to infuse the person- ality and be expressed in constructive ways.

The 1960s also saw the emergence of a strong feminist movement, which has led to women becoming more assertive in claiming their rights and changing their role in society. Women are no longer so dependent on men. Men are no longer the sole providers or protectors of the family. This and the high divorce rate have had a significant impact on the psycho- logical and physical health of men. Embedded in the national psyche is the idea that women are more vulnerable, more needy, more likely to be victims, than men. It is a stereotype that ignores the obvious fact that men are experiencing more distress than ever before, as more families break up and more men are written out of the employment script. It is a stereotype that can make it difficult for men to get their distress acknowledged and their needs met.

Men who have not found a place in society, who have no concept of what it is to be a man, are vulnerable to a desperate sense of alienation, apathy and depression, which is reflected in the increasing suicide rates for young men. Perhaps what is missing most from the lives of many men is the positive presence of a father. There is a need for elders and mentors in the development of masculinity. What it is to be a man can only be learnt from other men, from their example and from their stories.

Dean's story *(Theme: sexually abused adult males)*
Dean is a 27-year-old man who was first referred to the mental health services five years ago following an attempt to hang him- self. He was found to be depressed and experiencing psychotic symptoms. He had a history of drug and alcohol misuse, criminal activity and promiscuous, abusive relationships with women. Since that time he has experienced frequent crises during which

intense feelings of anxiety and despair and persecutory ideas of a religious nature overwhelm him.

His father abandoned the family when Dean was three and he has had little contact with him since. His mother remarried, but that marriage broke down because of her husband's recidivism, when Dean was 11 years old. There were two children, both girls, from that relationship. His mother's behaviour towards him became sexualized at around this time. She began inviting Dean into her bed to keep her company because of her loneliness. At first it seemed to Dean an expression of her need for comfort, but it soon developed into sexualized contact, although stopping short of penetrative sex. Dean felt confused by his feelings; he knew that what was happening was wrong, but he also felt excited and aroused. When he refused, his mother denied that her conduct was seductive or coercive or in any way improper, instead accusing him of being 'over-sexed and dirty minded'. Dean did not see himself as a victim of abuse. The image he had grown up with was of women as the weaker sex, over whom men had power and responsibility. During the absence of his step-father Dean had been his mother's 'little man'. To see himself as a victim would be to undermine his sense of masculinity and to cast his mother in the role of an abuser. As Dean put it, 'She was my mother, there was no force, so how could it be abuse.'

Recovery work

Overcoming the destructive emotional legacy of abuse is likely to be long-term work. Dean found it easier to relate to a female because of his fears about being criticized by another man. He had previously disclosed his experience to a male probation officer who had advised him that such things were best forgotten. It was important that his story was accepted, although he presented it in a way that cast him in the role of a predatory male. Gradually, he began to acknowledge that as a young adolescent, his mother was more powerful than he was and that it was she who was responsible for upholding the incest taboo. It was important for Dean to understand that his arousal during the abuse was the autonomic response of a healthy body and did not signify any moral responsibility. As he began to identify himself as a victim and then more comfortably ally himself with a survivor role, his feelings of anger, fear, guilt and badness began to surface. The recovery work did not proceed smoothly. There were further crises involving acts of self-harm, drug taking and drinking. The work was further interrupted by flights into wellness and abrupt angry 'endings', in which Dean accused the worker of 'fucking up his mind'. Gradually the experience became a memory of pain rather than a painful memory.

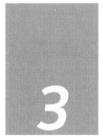

3 Creative solutions to crisis

Crisis intervention involves brief periods of intensive support aimed at helping people through periods of high levels of distress. If early signs of increasing distress are recognized and promptly and effectively responded to, an individual can be prevented from spiralling down into a deeply troubled and troubling state of mind that may lead to a psychiatric emergency. In this sense, crisis work may be seen as preventative. From the service user's perspective, a crisis is always a frightening experience and it is the responsibility of mental health services to support people through these chaotic periods in the most sensitive and effective way possible, minimizing further distress, risk and loss of liberty (Minghella *et al.,* 1998).

Crises can occur for many reasons. They commonly occur at times of transition, either developmental, situational or both, when the challenges of living overwhelm or exhaust our resources. How well we cope with the challenges of living depends on three factors:

- The nature of the challenge. The meaning it has for us. The magnitude and predictability of it and the amount of control we have.
- The resources we have to draw on. Our personal coping strategies and the support we have available.
- Our sense of personal agency, of being in control of our lives.

Caplan (1964), in his seminal work on crisis theory, proposed that crisis should not be seen as illness or inadequacy but as a potential turning point in an individual's life. Although a crisis is a painful and disorganizing experience, it is also an opportunity to learn something helpful about our lives and ourselves. It is an experience from which many people emerge stronger and more integrated. For people with a vulnerability to severely disorganizing distress, a crisis can be a frightening, demoralizing experience for which many seek relief in medication and admission. To seek resolution solely through the sanctuary and support of a hospital admission and through the use of medication, can limit the opportunity to learn how to be more resourceful in managing future episodes of distress in a way that reduces the tendency to spiral out of control. Frequent crises can also be demoralizing for mental health professionals who begin to blame themselves, or the client, or colleagues, and feel powerless to change the relapse/readmission cycle. If both staff and client could see crisis as an opportunity to learn how to manage the problems of living more effectively, then breakdown becomes an opportunity for breakthrough and crisis can be viewed more positively.

Some clinicians argue that we should also recognize that a crisis is not a turning point that leads to change for everyone. Some people remain highly vulnerable to troubled states of mind and periods of well-being seem fragile and transient. Such individuals need high levels of ongoing support as part of a carefully orchestrated care plan. This should include a crisis plan that aims to prevent the development of crisis episodes where possible and minimize distress and disruption where it is not.

Caplan identified phases in the development of a crisis that individuals pass through (Figure 3.1). Resolution can occur at any stage if people are:

- Able to discover the resourcefulness to bring about some change in the precipitating events.
- Bring about some change in the way they perceive those events.
- Bring about some change in the way they react.

People unknown to the mental health services may reach the third stage before they are referred. For those with a known vulnerability and a history of contact with the service this may happen at an earlier stage. We all have

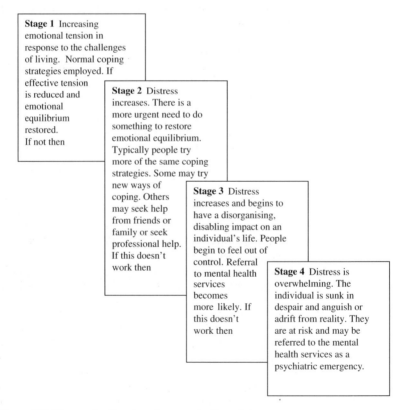

Figure 3.1 Stages in the development of a crisis

our own stress reaction pattern and express vulnerability in individual ways. For some people that reaction can be quite disabling and sometimes catastrophic in which they spiral down into deep despair or enter a confusing and threatening reality.

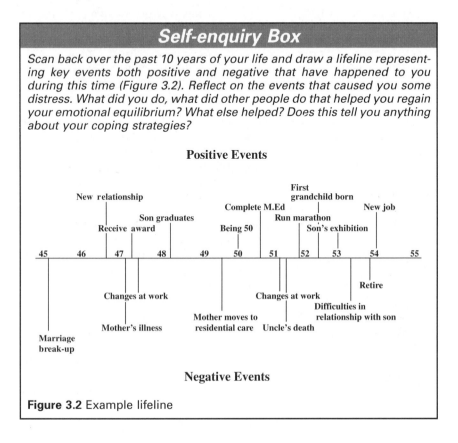

Self-enquiry Box

Scan back over the past 10 years of your life and draw a lifeline representing key events both positive and negative that have happened to you during this time (Figure 3.2). Reflect on the events that caused you some distress. What did you do, what did other people do that helped you regain your emotional equilibrium? What else helped? Does this tell you anything about your coping strategies?

Positive Events

Negative Events

Figure 3.2 Example lifeline

Early intervention

Many people are extremely fearful of relapse and show a strong interest in learning about early warning signs (McDermott, 1998). In fact, many vulnerable people and their carers become knowledgeably aware of signs of relapse without any help from mental health professionals. Relapse increases the probability of further crises and the likelihood of persistent disability and social dislocation (Birchwood and Tarrier, 1994). Also it leaves people feeling demoralized and lacking control over their lives. The early signs scale developed by Birchwood *et al.* is a widely used, reliable assessment tool for helping clients, their carers and mental health professionals to identify a client's relapse signature and monitor early signs that precede episodes of disruptive distress. Signs that typically resemble anxiety and depression are frequently the earliest indicators, followed by the gradual emergence of uninhibited behaviour and intrusive, troubling thoughts.

Frequently reported early signs

Feeling low	Losing one's temper easily
Difficulty in managing everyday tasks and interactions	Being very excitable
	Feeling confused or puzzled
Feeling useless or helpless	Feeling of being talked about
Feeling dissatisfied with self	or laughed at
Difficulty in concentrating	Talking or acting in
Feeling tense, afraid or anxious	inappropriate ways
Feeling irritable	Feeling of being watched
Restless, unsatisfying sleep	Talking or smiling to self

A number of services in the UK have developed client-held documents that outline relapse signatures, coping strategies and the interventions that help. All mental health service users with complex problems are legally entitled to a coordinated care programme that should include early warning signs and a collaboratively developed crisis plan. The cognitive, emotional and behavioural characteristics of a person's relapse signature can be recorded in explicit straightforward language rather than technical terminology. Describing an early sign as 'a slowing down of speech, thought and action', is more helpful than 'increasing psychomotor retardation', 'being bothered by thoughts that people are able to see into my mind' is better than 'an increase in intrusive paranoid thinking'. Relapse prevention plans should also include information about trigger events.

Common triggers include:

- Conflicts within family relationships and conflicts with others.
- Excessive psycho-social stimulus, which can sometimes occur as a consequence of the unrealistic expectations of professional helpers and others.
- Loss of key relationships, including the actual or anticipated withdrawal of support from mental health professionals.
- Lack of a meaningful way of structuring time.
- Social isolation.
- Social disadvantage and oppression.
- Stopping medication.
- Use of recreational drugs.

Sometimes clients are able to quantify the strength of relapse signs on a simple rating scale. For example, 'On a scale of 1–10, where 10 is the worst this anxious preoccupation with what people might be thinking about you has been, where would you put yourself at the moment?' Continued monitoring can be a helpful indicator not only of severity but also of the time scale involved in an individual's relapse pattern. Some people spiral down very quickly into a distressed and chaotic state in a matter of days, whereas others might be able to maintain a higher level of functioning for several weeks before a deterioration begins to impact disruptively on their lives. A relapse prevention plan that includes early signs monitoring is essential for people who want to try living without long-term medication or want to reduce it and avoid a further disruptive breakdown in their personal and social functioning. However, relapse monitoring is not appropriate or help-ful for every client. Birchwood comments that for some clients the repetitive requests for information may increase anxiety about relapse and over-emphasize the psychiatric vulnerability. Monitoring will also be difficult with those who have limited or fluctuating insight. It is often not practical to use systematic monitoring continuously, but it can be helpfully intro-duced during periods of stress or when the first early signs become evident. Mental health professionals who have worked closely with a service user, sometimes over several years, get to know an individual's early signs pat-tern, which can be quite idiosyncratic. Carers, too, will often be aware of subtle but significant early signs of relapse and justifiably complain that these observations have not always been taken seriously and responded to by mental health professionals.

Naomi's story *(Theme: early signs monitoring)*
Mark, my son, first became ill when he was nineteen. We noticed that he had become very quiet over a period of several weeks, he seemed distant and distracted as if he had got something on his mind. We thought he must be worrying about something, but he just got irritable if we asked what was bothering him, in fact he became quite abusive at times, which was so unlike him. I won-dered if he was still getting over breaking up with his girlfriend or if he was upset because his father had recently re-married and moved to live closer to his work. I made him go to the doctor who said she thought Mark was depressed and prescribed some antidepressants. After I suppose about 3 months he virtually stopped going out socially and was missing more and more of his college course. He began to do odd things like wearing sun-glasses in the house or turning his head away from people when they spoke to him or passed him in the street. Often he would sleep late and be wandering about the house at night. One night I heard him crying and went down to him. He told me that certain people on the television were able to see right into his mind and that when people stared at him in the street they knew that he was different. He was also hearing voices telling him that he had 'gone wrong' and would have to be 'dealt with'. When we tried to talk to him about it the next day he just got very excitable and aggressive. We had to call the doctor and a social worker and he was admitted to hospital. I suppose it must have been about 4 months from the time we first became concerned about him till he was admitted and we were told he was suffering from schizophrenia. It was such a traumatic time. We couldn't accept it at first. No one in either of our families had had psychiatric problems and up until that time Mark had seemed just a normal young man.
This was six years ago and since then he has had two more admissions. We are hoping now that Mark is taking a newer drug with fewer side-effects, that he'll continue taking them and will stay well. The other positive and helpful part of his recent care has been

that he has been able to forge a good relationship with his CPN, who monitors Mark quite closely, though not in an intrusive way, for early signs that he is breaking down again. We know what to look for now and I think Mark himself recognizes when things are beginning to go wrong. Sunglasses or shutting or blinking his eyes a lot are a sign. He seems low in spirits at these times and stands around in a rather pensive preoccupied sort of way and is reluctant to go out. When we notice this we know it won't be long before Mark begins to be troubled by voices and the idea that people can see what he calls his 'impurity'. He does become quite distressed when he reaches this stage. What seems to help is being in quiet surroundings. Working in the garden or taking the dogs for a walk also seems to help. If he's around a lot of people he seems more troubled. His psychiatrist usually increases his medication and his CPN comes in more regularly and talks to him about his worrying thoughts and any current problems he has. It's difficult to know exactly what triggers off these unsettled episodes. Usually it's something to do with him feeling left behind, seeing others getting on with their lives – building careers, setting up home, getting married and having children. In many ways he is still an adolescent with all the anxieties and insecurities about finding a place in the adult world.

Crisis services

Wood (1994) in a consideration of over 40 reports on the views of users found strong support for a community-based crisis service that offered an alternative to admission. Some admissions to a hospital setting will continue to be necessary. They have positive outcomes for many people, providing 'time out', access to intensive support and a milieu in which distress can be contained and reduced. But studies indicate the length of stay for many is much longer than needed, mainly because of a lack of accommodation and home-based support and that 40% of those treated in acute wards will be readmitted within a year (Sainsbury Centre, 1998b).

The Sainsbury Centre survey found that much of the current inpatient care that people have access to is 'anti-therapeutic'. It often does not address individuals' psycho-social needs, even though these factors underlie the crisis. The care programmes may become routinized and limited, lacking in therapeutic focus, rather than individualized and responsive to assessed and expressed need. Surveys of the experience of service users admitted to acute wards highlight the lack of meaningful activity, the absence of a relaxed environment in which they feel safe and supported, poor amenities and limited one-to-one contact with ward staff. Women in particular expressed dissatisfaction with issues of safety and privacy (Mental Health Act Commission, 1997; Sainsbury Centre, 1998b).

It is now widely recognized that some crisis care can be delivered to people in their own homes or in crisis houses that can provide sanctuary and skilled support. While credible community-based crisis services have been slow to develop in the UK, the evidence base demonstrating their effectiveness is growing (Dean and Gadd, 1990; Burns *et al.*, 1993; Minghella *et al.*, 1998). In response to local need, community-orientated crisis services with different configurations have emerged in the UK. They involve some of the following residential and non-residential services:

- Crisis houses
- Sanctuaries/respite accommodation
- Supported housing
- Community Mental Health Teams providing an extended hours crisis service
- Home treatment teams/crisis intervention teams providing an extended hours service
- Assertive outreach teams providing an extended hours service
- Drop in centres
- Mental health resource centres
- Counselling services
- Telephone crisis lines
- Carer support and family consultation
- Family 'adoption'
- Psychiatric triage in Accident and Emergency departments
- Crisis companions/befrienders.

It is often the fear of being hospitalized, of being medicated, of being sectioned and the stigma and loss of autonomy that that entails, which prevents people seeking help in the early stages of a crisis. Crisis services therefore need to address these issues. Crisis houses should provide a safe, supportive environment in which people can take 'time out' to recover and learn from their crisis. They need to provide accessible one-to-one contact with staff and opportunities for recuperative solitude. Some crisis houses have been set up for women only. These create an environment free from harassment, where gender-related issues, which are often precipitating factors, can be shared, respected and understood (Wakelin, 1998). Skallagrigg House in Birmingham and Drayton Park in London are examples of women-only crisis houses that provide a safe environment in which the process of recovery from severe mental health problems, based on resourceful self-management, can begin. Other services have developed in response to the mental health needs of ethnic minority groups. An excellent example of this is KUSH, a black sanctuary and crisis outreach team in Hackney, London that offers a rapid response service to the African-Caribbean community (Wakelin, 1997). Assessment is holistic, early diagnosis is avoided and crisis is understood in the context of people's lives. Intervention is in the form of practical help, information, counselling addressing ethnicity, gender and faith issues, the arts therapies and complementary therapies. Medication is always an option, but is not central to the therapeutic approach. The aim is to encourage a more positive attitude towards the mental health services among people from the black community with severe and enduring mental health problems, many of whom may have had abusive experiences of psychiatry in the past.

Crisis management

The immediate task in crisis management is to intervene in a way that brings a sense of safety and containment to the situation and reduces the level of distress. People caught up in escalating distress often feel troubled, helpless and out of control. It is important to act calmly, to listen, and to be a supportive presence. If people are not too disturbed by an experience of a confused and threatening reality, or too sunk in despair or too fearful and agitated, it is usually possible to engage them in conversation about their distress. As they begin to talk about their experience, the flow of words carries and dissipates some of the emotional pain and tension. The cathartic expression of feeling in appropriate ways can be experienced as a release and a relief. Being heard in an empathic way anchors the client psychologically in calmer waters. Where people are too distracted by their distress or too sunk in their despair to engage in conversation, it is important to try to be an undemanding compassionate presence, leaving people feeling cared for and held psychologically.

Once some of the intensity has diminished, it is possible to engage people in problem solving in relation to events surrounding the crisis. Gerard Egan's problem management model of helping, (discussed in Part 2), offers a framework for approaching this task in a systematic way. Within the context of a problem-solving process, it may be possible for people to take some action to change the circumstances that have led to the development of the crisis. Secondly, it may be possible for them perceive the situation differently so that it becomes less problematic. Finally, the client may be able to change their reaction to events so that they become less distressing (Figure 3.3). Through engaging in supported problem-solving to manage the challenges of everyday living, clients gradually internalize this skill and learn to be more resourceful and less crisis prone.

Of crucial importance in the management of a crisis is the level of social support to which a person has access. The recurrent and disturbing nature of a severely troubled state of mind results in many people becoming isolated from the broad stream of social life and lacking the emotional and practical support of family and friends. They become attached to professional helpers as their main source of support. A therapeutic system forms, within which a service user seeks to meet their dependency needs. Like family systems, therapeutic systems may not always provide an emotional climate that is conducive to recovery and well-being. In fact it may be the system that holds the individual in a 'sick role', if support is given in an intrusive, imposing way or given conditionally. The system then becomes part of the problem rather than the solution. The development of self-help groups and user-run services, independent advocacy and volunteer befriending schemes are significant attempts to de-professionalize support and put caring back into the community. Many people are, of course, supported with great love and care by their families who often feel unsupported themselves by professional services.

Strategies for changing

The situation

Noticing and reducing the influence of triggers; supported problem-solving; practical help with pressing social issues; conflict management; family consultation and carer support; solution focused interventions; mobilizing social support; accessible/available professional support; respite care; inpatient care.

The perception

Re-evaluation of experience through cognitive strategies and other therapeutic approaches; dialogue that supportively challenges and raises awareness; crisis as a living-learning experience; information/education; encouraging realistic hopefulness; encouraging a sense of mastery over the challenges of living.

The reaction

Coping strategies enhancement; early signs monitoring and early intervention; response inhibition and wise action; verbalizing concerns and appropriately discharging feelings; relaxation techniques; guided visualization; religious support and spiritual sustenance; complementary therapies; medication; self-soothing; restorative self-care; risk management; defusing aggression.

Figure 3.3 Crisis management

Self-enquiry Box

You may find it helpful to revisit a scene from your own crisis work. Take a few moments to settle and quieten yourself. Bring to mind a scenario from your practice that left you feeling dissatisfied.

Replay the scene

Where did this interaction take place?
Who was there?
What did the client do or say?
What did you do or say?
What happened next?
What was the outcome?
How did that leave you feeling?
What would you have done differently?
How do you imagine the outcome would have differed?

Run it again

This time visualize yourself intervening in a different way that leads to your preferred outcome.
    You may find it useful to use this structure within the context of supervision.

Justine's story

Justine is a 35-year-old British born African-Caribbean woman who has been referred to the acute psychiatric inpatient services on eighteen occasions over the past 15 years. The usual scenario is that she becomes increasingly excitable and caught up in a web of unusual thoughts, both of an egotistical and persecutory nature. Before too long there is a hostile confrontation with a member of the public, the police become involved and she is admitted under a section of the Mental Health Act. Admission is resented and resisted and usually exacerbates Justine's distress and delusional thinking. She frequently refuses antipsychotic drugs and, because of her highly aroused hostile behaviour, is given her medication by injection. After about a week Justine is usually more composed and less immersed in her delusional world, although she remains volatile and very sensitive to the behaviour of staff towards her. Periods of admission have lasted between three weeks and three months, during which time Justine becomes a subdued and compliant figure.

Justine is divorced and has a child who lives with her ex-husband and his wife. She has not held a job for 10 years and lives by herself in a council flat. Her main source of support is her mother. Unfortunately, this support takes an unhelpful form when Justine is unwell. She sees her daughter's behaviour as 'the devil having hold of her tongue' and has on occasions brought members of her local Pentecostal church to visit Justine to 'heal her through prayer'. Justine does not share her mother's faith and finds these healing invocations upsetting. She is desperate for another relationship and often she has become involved in sexually and financially exploitative relationships with men she has picked up in local pubs and clubs.

Justine has a negative view of herself, both as a person and as a woman. She often feels isolated and lonely and excluded from the mainstream of life. She feels stigmatized by her psychiatric history and, as a consequence, is not very receptive to the idea of becoming a member of a local resource centre for people with long-term mental health problems. She does have frequent contact with a CPN and a support worker, who also has an African-Caribbean background. It is her frequent ruminations on what's missing from her life and her frustrated attempts to claim an ordinary life for herself that seem to precipitate a crisis spiral. An early sign is that she expresses more dissatisfaction and despondency with herself and her life and becomes irritable and is easily angered. She then rapidly spirals from a low mood into excitable chaotic behaviour and, before long, delusional beliefs begin to emerge. She believes that she is a reincarnation of an African Princess and that her daughter is also of royal blood. She says she has been reborn in exile to be safe from 'all the killing' and that she receives messages in news reports on television. Often she will behave unwisely, giving all her clothes and belongings to Oxfam or buying expensive jewellery for her daughter.

The staff team involved in Justine's care have established a crisis plan with her in an attempt to minimize the distress and disruption of crisis episodes and reduce the need for such frequent admissions. Justine holds a copy of this plan.

Crisis plan

- Be aware of early signs.
- Increase support. Daily contact with CPN and support worker.
- Work on here and now feelings and frustrations, including gender and ethnicity issues.
- Strengthen self-esteem/feel more positive about myself/make use of personal history book.
- Hold on to hopefulness.
- Avoid demanding, over-stimulating social situations/precipitating events.
- Get appropriate support from mother.
- Make use of self-coping strategies.
- Increase medication.

If feeling more troubled, excitable and delusional I would prefer the following plan to be implemented:

- Seek bed in The Willows (crisis house).
- Engage in quiet activity with staff.
- Frequent opportunity for conversation with staff, focusing on here and now feelings and frustration.
- Opportunity to talk about my unusual beliefs and minimize adverse consequences or unwise action associated with those beliefs.
- Aromatherapy massage.
- Art therapy.
- Maintain medication programme.
- Learn from the crisis experience, incorporate learning into my repertoire of coping skills.

Risk assessment and management

Risk is high on the agenda of mental health services. The recent spate of high profile inquiries into acts of homicide committed by people with known mental health problems, has raised public fears about the safety of care in the community policies. In fact, the incidence of violence towards others is low compared with acts of suicide and self-harm. The continuing problem of caring for at-risk clients in the community has been the subject of a number of reports, most notably the Richie Report (1994). These all point to inadequate communication and liaison between the various agencies involved;

inadequacies in gathering a full, accurate, verified history; Section 117 after-care procedures not being closely followed; a failure to adopt an assertive outreach approach to the delivery of care, or respond to early warning signs of a relapse and, last but not least, a neglect of the rule that the best predictor of future behaviour is past behaviour. The result is the inadequate delivery of care to individuals involved with the inevitable tragic consequences. While all risk will never be eliminated in mental health care, there is clearly a need for continuing scrutiny of risk assessment and management procedures and processes.

Risk is generally defined as the likelihood of an adverse event happening. In a psychiatric context it refers to:

- Harm to others.
- Harm to self.
- Neglect of self.
- Exploitation by others.

Not all risk should be considered adverse. However, in a climate of criticism and blame, mental health services tend to retreat into defensive practice. A cornerstone of the humanistic philosophy of care is the right of the client to self-determination and the dignity of risk but, in the prevailing climate, there is a very real danger of overly cautious, restrictive care practices being adopted. Harrison (1997) argues that rather than trying to eliminate risk we should see some risk-taking as part of the process of enabling people to re-engage in life. Morgan (1998) draws attention to the fact that for most service users with a history of vulnerability to severely troubled states of mind, the community poses bigger threats than users do to themselves and others. Many service users experience:

- Abuse and hostility from the public.
- Sexual abuse and exploitation.
- Domestic violence.
- Homelessness.
- Poverty.
- Social exclusion, isolation and loneliness.
- Relapse.
- Lack of socially valued occupational/recreational opportunities.
- Involvement with the police criminal justice system.

Assessment of risk is a continuous process. The daily care of clients involves making choices and decisions that will involve some element of risk. Risk assessment should be explicitly open and always involve the client and carers. For some individuals, particularly those who have a known history of risk behaviour or whose history reveals significant risk factors, a more systematic assessment might be required. This may be carried out and repeated as part of a care programme approach under Section 117 of the Mental Health Act.

Risk factors in aggression and violence
- A previous history of violence.
- A diagnosis of schizophrenia with paranoid features.
- Signs of a relapse.
- Presence of positive symptoms such as delusions of persecution and command hallucinations.
- Outbursts of anger.
- Drug and/or alcohol misuse.
- Deterioration in social/family relationships.
- Threats of violence/declared intentions.
- Loss of contact with the mental health services.
- Non-adherence to medication programme.
- Developmental history of exposure to aggression and violence.
- Cultural values in relation to aggression and violent acts.
- Failure to learn to delay gratification of wants.
- Inability to cope with frustration and conflicts.
- Failure to learn alternative strategies, other than aggression.
- Unresolved conflicts.
- Impulsive behaviour.
- Hostility to authority.
- Preoccupation with violent fantasies.
- Denial of aggressive behaviour.
- Lack of remorse.

(Adapted from Morgan, 1998)

Self-enquiry Box

You may find it helpful to reflect on a client with whom you are currently working, who has a history of exhibiting aggressive or violent behaviour, who may or may not have been involved in a formal risk assessment. Identify how many of the risk factors outlined above apply to this person. Are there others not listed?

If it seems appropriate, discuss with the person concerned their experience of managing their aggressive and violent tendencies. The following questions are offered as a guide, but you will probably want to reframe them to suit your own conversational style and the client involved.

'Are there times now, or have there been in the past, when you've had thoughts of harming others?'
'How often do you have those kind of thoughts?'
'Have there been occasions when you've acted on those thoughts?'
'What did you do?'
'What happened to the person involved?'
'What's prevented you from acting on those thoughts?'
'Have the police ever been involved?'
'Are there certain situations in which you find yourself becoming angry and have an impulse to behave aggressively or violently?'
'When was the last time. Could you describe what happened?'
'What is it about these situations that causes you to react in that way?'
'Had you been drinking or taking drugs at the time?'

> *'Have there been times when you've reacted differently?'*
> *'Could you imagine yourself dealing with that situation differently, dealing with your feelings without behaving aggressively or violently?'*
> *'On a scale of 1–10, how worried should I be about you harming others over the next week?'*

A more immediate assessment of risk will, of course, be necessary when a client is in an aroused and hostile state of mind. The degree of arousal and control can be assessed from the client's non-verbal behaviour, such as muscular tension, agitation, invading personal space, hostile silence or loud aggressive tone of speech and from verbal threats, abusive language and destructive acts to property. They may or may not be responsive to defusing, calming interventions. This should be seen as an early indication of the likely course of events, either towards regaining composure or towards an escalation of hostility. This latter scenario, particularly if in conjunction with some of the above risk factors, would signify a challenging situation in which there was potentially an immediate risk to the safety of others.

Dealing with anger and hostile behaviour

- Acknowledge the person's anger and their right to their feelings.
- Allow the expression of anger in appropriate safe ways – verbalizing anger, discharge of anger in non-destructive acts. Anger is self-limiting unless restimulated.
- Try and stay calm (use self-coaching and relaxation techniques). Provide psychological containment. Stay in the 'same gear', avoid any tendency to retaliate or appease.
- Be aware of your body language. Try not to communicate threatening non-verbal signals.
- Don't try to defend the situation or individuals the person is angry about.
- Avoid a struggle of wills, somebody has to lose. Look for compromise.
- Be aware of power issues in the helping relationship and a person's need to rebel, or the need to reclaim power and assert autonomy.
- Set limits. Encourage self-restraint. Raise awareness of response cost.
- Help the person explore the immediate cause of their anger.
- Help the client to engage in problem-solving. Be clear about what you can and cannot do.
- Accept that some anger may be projected or displaced on to you.
- Don't take unnecessary risks. Be aware of the indicators of high risk. If a person's anger is not subsiding but is in danger of escalating into destructive or violent acts, take whatever action is necessary to protect yourself and others.
- Debrief with colleagues after the incident. Decide if you need any additional support.

Risk factors in suicide
- Gender (more females attempt, more males succeed).
- Age – higher rates with increasing age.
- Cultural component (Asian women, young males).
- Marital status (higher in single, widowed, separated, divorced).
- Strength of emotional ties with others.
- Unemployment.
- Family history of suicide.
- Limited social support system.
- Experience of social exclusion/sense of alienation.
- Recent problematic life events.
- History of previous suicide attempts.
- Diagnosis of depression, manic depressive disorder or schizophrenia.
- Serious or terminal physical illness.
- Alcohol and/or drug misuse.
- Sleep disorder.
- Expressed intent.
- Evidence of planning.
- Evidence of preparation.
- Access to the means.
- Recovery phase in severe depression.
- Recent discharge from hospital.
- Expression of hopelessness.
- Development of trusting relationship with helpers and optimism about the efficacy of treatment and care.

(Adapted from Morgan, 1998)

There is an important distinction between suicidal behaviour and self-harm behaviour. In the latter the motivation is other than the wish to die, although it is true that some people who self-harm seem ambivalent about the outcome or unconcerned about the consequences. Self-harm behaviour is a coping strategy – albeit a damaging and potentially dangerous one, a means of gaining some relief from distress. Often what underlies self-harm behaviour is the desire to punish self or others, to draw attention to psychological pain or to gain relief from emotional tension. People who self-harm often experience antipathy, if not openly critical and judgemental attitudes, from professional helpers, who see their often repeated acts of self-injury as consciously manipulative and attention seeking. Self-mutilation and self-poisoning produce strong emotional reactions in professional helpers. Staff may feel baffled, helpless, let down, guilty, angry, horrified, fearful and sad in response to an individual's persistent self-harm. Once established as a distress relief pattern, some forms of self-harm, such as cutting, can be a difficult habit to break. Until some other strategy for coping with the emotional pain is found or the underlying emotional issues or current problems are less pressing, self-harm remains for many clients a means of survival or, as Arnold (1995) puts it, a way of bearing what would otherwise be unbearable.

Risk factors in self-harm
- Young people (15–25).
- Women are twice as likely as men to self-harm.
- Social deprivation.
- Emotional discord in significant relationships.
- Previous history of acts of self-harm.
- Drug and/or alcohol misuse.
- Sexual abuse in childhood.
- Emotional or physical abuse.
- Parental neglect.
- Parental loss.
- Rape or sexual abuse as an adult.
- Domestic violence.
- Lack of emotionally supportive relationships.
- Loss of a child or inability to have children.
- Emotional overwhelm.
- Self-hatred/low self-esteem.
- Intense feelings of anger/ anxiety.
- Powerlessness.
- Neediness.
- Dissociation/numbness/experience of unreality.

(Source: Arnold, 1995)

Self-enquiry Box

You may find it helpful to reflect on a client with whom you are currently working who has:
A history of attempted suicide or is considered to be at risk
or
A history of self-harm behaviour.
Identify how many of the risk factors outlined above apply to this person. Are there others not listed?
If it seems appropriate, discuss with the person concerned their experience of feeling suicidal or their need to self-harm and the way they express or manage those tendencies. The following questions are offered as a guide, but you will probably want to re-frame them to suit your own conversational style and the client concerned.
'Have you harmed yourself/attempted to end your life at any time in the past?'
'How do you feel about what happened?'
'Do you have thoughts of harming yourself/ending your life now?'
'Have you thought about how you might do that?'
'Do you have the means to do that?'
'When you think about harming yourself/ending your life, do you consider doing it where you won't be discovered?'
'How often do you have these thoughts?'
'What's stopped you acting on these thoughts?'
'On a scale of 1–10, how likely is that you will end your life?'
'Have there been times recently when you've felt it's worth carrying on living?'

'Could you describe the feeling you get when you experience a need to self-harm?'
'If you could draw it/paint it what would it look like?'
'When you experience this need to harm yourself are you able to resist it?'
'Are you aware of the risks you take when you self-harm?'
What's the feeling you get after you've harmed yourself?'
'Do you talk about these thoughts to anyone?'
'Do you know why you feel like harming yourself/ending your life?'
'On a scale of 1–10, how bad are these problems that make you want to end your life?'
'Are there others ways of getting relief/some peace without ending your life?'
What's helped you to keep on going till now, despite it being so bad?'
'What was happening in your life when these thoughts started?'
'What would you do if these thoughts of harming yourself/ending your life recur?'
'On a scale of 1–10, with 10 being very concerned and 1 being no concern at all, how concerned, should I be about you harming yourself/attempting to end your life over the next 24 hours?'
'How realistic is it of me to expect you to stay safe over the weekend?'
'On a scale of 1–10, where 10 is feeling very safe, what would that look like?
Who would be around? What would be happening?'

Annie's story *(Theme: managing the risk of suicide)*
Annie is a woman, aged 43, who has a history of depression and who has recently attempted suicide by asphyxiation with a neck ligature. She is divorced and lives with her two children, a boy aged 20 and a girl aged 17. Six months ago her mother died.

Shirley is a CPN working with a crisis service and has been caring for Annie since her discharge from the acute admission ward 2 weeks ago.

I'd been depressed on and off for about 10 years. More or less since I left my husband. I didn't have a very happy marriage. He used to drink a lot and knock me about and half strangle me. I thought that I would feel a lot better about my life and myself after I left him. I've been on all sorts of antidepressants but they haven't really lifted my depression, just stopped me feeling so desperate. Depression is difficult to explain. Most of the time it's like living in shadow – you can never find a place in the sun. But sometimes the shadows seem to darken and you feel as if you've done something terribly wrong and something dreadful is going to happen to you. Once before when I felt that way, I took an overdose, but more to get some relief than anything else. A few weeks ago my daughter said to me, 'You're such a drudge Mum, when are you going to get a life? It sort of hit me how bleak and empty my life had become. I suppose I'm afraid of life. I tend to see disasters behind every door. So I don't open any, don't take any risks. About a week before this happened I was staring at myself in the mirror and I heard my mother's voice saying, 'You'll never amount to anything. Get out of my sight.' I was frightened that I was going mad. After that I couldn't get this thought out of my head that I should get out of everybody's sight. I thought it all out. I picked a night when my children were out and wouldn't be back till late and wouldn't miss me until the morning, then drove to the coast. I knew I wanted to die by the sea.

Shirley's story
I've known Annie about 2 weeks now. She was discharged from hospital after 10 days' close observation. There are some risks and I am quite concerned about her safety, but her experience of hospital was not particularly helpful in reducing her distress. What helps me to deal with my anxiety about her care is being clear about my responsibilities and having the support and involvement of the multidisciplinary crisis team. She is still quite depressed and some days feels unable to go on. We have given her quite a bit of responsibility for herself. I assess the level of risk regularly and trust her to be open with me about her suicidal thoughts. I ask her how concerned I should be about her during the next 24 hours and how safe she feels. I'm getting to know when she's having a bad day, her face has this haunted look and her voice loses its power and becomes almost a whisper. I'm meeting with her four days a week at the moment. We also have an arrangement where she will phone the service if she's feeling at risk and I or someone will call and spend some time with her, or talk on the phone, then if she is still feeling unsafe she goes to a friend's house or to Beacon House (crisis house). We've also been looking at ways of managing her bad days so that she's not so vulnerable to her depressive thoughts and feelings. I think she was shocked by the frightened, angry reaction of her children to her suicide attempt. She feels guilty about upsetting her children so much and not wanting to put them through that again has given her a reason to go on living at the moment. The children are still quite angry with her and some of my work has involved helping them deal with their feelings and help them not to feel burdened by responsibility for their mother's safety. Also I think it has been a relief to be able to talk about some of the here and now difficulties in her life and I sense she is beginning to feel a little more hopeful about the future, perhaps seeing this crisis as a turning point. I've begun to engage her in some problem solving around her relationship with her children. Also there were some house repairs that needed urgent attention and were a worry and I've been able to help her with those. Annie has experienced a lot of trauma in her life. Her mother wasn't able to give her much affection or approval and was quite harsh with Annie because of her enuresis, sometimes shutting her in the cupboard under the stairs as a punishment. Annie's also had a violent marriage which further undermined her self-esteem. She

> has agreed to explore some of these earlier traumas with a clinical psychologist. She has shown a lot of courage in her life – leaving her husband, bringing up the children by herself and I'm hopeful she will be able to draw on this resolve in overcoming her depression.

Responding to self-harm and suicidal behaviour

Managing risk in the care of suicidal or self-harm clients is not just about intervening in restrictive, controlling ways in an attempt to eliminate opportunities. Sometimes strategies that rely too heavily on observation and control paradoxically increase the risk. A depressed and suicidal person's sense of worthlessness and hopelessness may be increased by a care regimen that emphasizes close or continuous observation, but neglects pressing psychosocial needs. Self-harm clients may take greater risks in harming themselves if their need to self-harm safely, in the absence of more constructive strategies for dealing with emotional tension, is not recognized. It is not possible to eliminate all risk even in a hospital setting. Ultimately, service users carry responsibility for their own decisions and actions. Engaging service users in collaborative assessment and care planning can open up the opportunity for 'positive risk taking' (Morgan and Hemming, 1999). This is not the negligent avoidance of professional responsibility for providing directive and restrictive care where a person is unsafe. It is care that respects the dignity of risk and the rights and responsibilities of individuals to confront the problems of living and to face the reality of human suffering within a supportive therapeutic system. Strategies that promote positive risk taking include:

- Engage in an open exploration of suicidal ideas – the frequency, intrusiveness, planning and motivation.
- Assess risk factors.
- Be present with clients in calm, accepting, empathic ways.
- Engage in therapeutic conversation that facilitates the safe discharge of distress and the identification of underlying issues and concerns.
- Recognize the opportunity for learning, growth and change in the crisis experience.
- Work collaboratively with at-risk clients and their family/carer in assessing needs and planning care.
- Negotiate a risk minimization plan with the client and their family/carer.
- Be clear about a person's responsibility for his or her own safety within the context of the plan.
- Accept that in the short term some self-harm may continue and a more immediate and realistic objective is minimal risk.
- Communicate the plan to all workers involved.
- Be clear about the availability of support when a person feels unsafe and the boundaries that apply.
- Mobilize social support.
- Engage in problem solving with client.

- Help maximize client's constructive coping strategies and develop others.
- Instil hope and realistic optimism.
- Be aware of your responsibility and accountability as a professional practitioner.
- Make use of support systems, supervision and training opportunities to maintain aware and responsive care.

Working with clients who represent a risk to themselves or others in positive risk-taking ways is challenging and exciting, but also anxiety provoking. To practise confidently, particularly within a culture of blame requires a cohesive framework of accountability and responsibility, linking practitioner, multidisciplinary team and organization. Where this is inadequately defined, defensive practice is likely to flourish.

A person-centred approach to assessment

4

By person-centred assessment I mean gathering information and understandings about a client's inner and outer worlds from their frame of reference. It should, as far as possible, be a collaborative process in which the helper and client try to identify what is going on and what is going wrong (and right too). As Egan (1994) puts it, it involves helping clients 'see what they don't see and need to see to make sense of their chaotic behaviour – all in the service of helping them manage their lives more effectively' (p. 143). Although an assessment interview may be a discrete event, building a picture of a client's world, their problems of living, their needs, their strengths, talents and resources, is often a continuing process that is interwoven with the process of recovery/change. Assessment rightly takes a holistic approach to understanding distress. How could we understand how someone has become sunk in despair, or a prisoner of their fears, or persecuted by voices unless we were prepared to be a compassionate presence in their search for meaning in the psychological, social, spiritual and bodily dimensions of their experience? But we need to approach this task with humility. To think that through an assessment process we could come to 'know' a person in all their complexity would be disrespectful arrogance. At best we can, through our conversations and our developing relationship, come to some shared understanding about their experience of suffering and the help they need.

There has in recent years been some recognition of the value of a strengths-orientated assessment process in mental health care (Morgan, 1993, 1996). Assessment that dwells too narrowly on an individual's problem-filled story is disempowering and undermines self-esteem and hopefulness. It can be much more helpful to focus on the strengths, skills, talents, resources, opportunities and aspirations than on problems, deficits and disabilities. Recovery is not about regaining a problem-free life – whose life is? It is about living life more resourcefully, living a satisfying and contributing life, in spite of limitations caused by a continuing vulnerability to disabling distress. Unless we see a person's strengths, qualities and talents, it is difficult to value them as individuals. The way we think about them and talk about them will have a negative slant. If we can nurture people's abilities, help them make the most of their strengths and support them in their interests and aspirations, they are more likely to be able to develop an identity not dominated by a psychiatric disability and claim an ordinary life for themselves.

Veterans of the psychiatric system often have a lot of interpersonal scarring and present in uncommunicative ways. Their message is 'I've been through all this before and I know what happens if I say too much'! Other clients will readily reveal symptoms, that is, express urgent needs in a psychiatric way in an interview with a mental health practitioner as a way of getting their needs met, at least partially. If the response is a routine psychiatric one – a change in medication, a prescriptive strategy or an admission, with no attempt made understand the distress pattern – then the experience of distress soon becomes mystified. In a short space of time a person is unable to recognize any connection between their thoughts, feelings and acts and the events in their lives. The further clients get into their psychiatric career the more difficult it becomes to unravel events past and present that have led to persistent disabilities or current crises (Mosher and Burti, 1994).

People seeking help from the mental health services often have complex problems of a personal, interpersonal and social nature – problems of living. They are often in contact with the services at times when they are experiencing considerable distress and psychological disturbance. More than anything else they need to engage in a dialogue with practitioners to reach some kind of shared definition of their situation and what should be done about it (Sheppard, 1993). Developing a dialogue in which people can *uncover* the problems of living they face; *discover* the meaning of disabling distress and begin the process of *recovery*, requires the skilled use of what Heron (1990) refers to as catalytic interventions. To my mind one of the most important catalytic skills is the ability to listen and to hear the other person. The experience and therapeutic value of being heard is eloquently captured by Carl Rogers in personal reflection:

I like being heard. A number of times in my life I have felt myself bursting with insoluble problems, or going round and round in tormented circles or, during one period being overcome by feelings of worthlessness and despair. I think I have been more fortunate than most in finding, at these times, individuals who have been able to hear me and thus rescue me from the chaos of my feelings, individuals who have been able to hear my meanings a little more deeply than I have known them. These persons have heard me without judging me, diagnosing me or evaluating me. They have just listened and clarified and responded to me at all the levels at which I was communicating. I can testify that when you are in psychological distress and someone really hears you without passing judgement on you, without trying to take responsibility for you, without trying to mould you, it feels damn good! At these times it has relaxed the tension in me. It has permitted me to bring out the frightening feelings, the guilt, the despair, the confusions that have been part of the experience. When I have been listened to and have been heard, I am able to perceive my world in a new way and go on. It is astonishing how elements that seem insoluble become soluble when someone listens, how confusions that seem irremediable turn into relatively clear flowing streams when one is heard. I have deeply appreciated the times that I have experienced this sensitive, empathic, concentrated listening of being heard. (Rogers, 1980 p. 12)

To listen well we need to have our attention free. This can so easily get caught up in our own needs and concerns or be difficult to sustain because our energy is low. We sometimes need to prepare ourselves to listen – to let go of other things and refocus our attention. I want to listen in an open way, not evaluating what the client says according to my own values; not trying to apply diagnostic criteria to their experience, but trying to understand it from their frame of reference. I want to try to be present with people in as relaxed and receptive way as I can. I want to tune in to the fullness of their experience and this means being receptive to what is communicated through non-verbal channels as well as linguistically. In other words, tuning in to what is not being said. It can be difficult to verbalize experience sometimes; everything seems confused or threatening and the client takes refuge from the reality of their situation behind a wall of inconsequential disclosures or withdrawal. Even though someone may say very little, their body language can communicate volumes. Emotional experience may be denied verbally, but leaks out authentically in expression, posture, movement and tone of voice.

Suggestions for improving listening

- Listening is hard work. It requires energy. It requires a commitment to listen well. It is difficult to listen if you are tired or if your own needs are pressing. Know what your limits are.
- Get physically prepared to listen. Make the environment as conducive as possible. Be aware of proximity and barriers. Check your body cues.
- Get mentally prepared to listen. Acknowledge distractions, personal or professional, put them to one side for attention later. Try to be aware of any assumptions, prejudice, stereotyping in relation to the client. Remind yourself that this is the client's time.
- Try to hold back on questions, interpretations, giving information and advice. Use a mental banking system of points to come back to. Trust yourself to ask the right question or find the right response, don't try to frame it while the client is talking. Be aware of the quality of silent interludes; wait receptively if they seem meaningful to the client.
- Try to avoid blocking tactics. 'I don't think I'm the best person to talk to'; ' I can't talk now, come and see me later'; 'Try not to worry about it'. Of course, at times, responding in these ways can be quite legitimate. Other blocking tactics include selective listening – hearing only what we want to hear; controlling the agenda by asking a series of questions; changing the subject; and using non-verbal cues to block the conversation.

There are a number of other catalytic interventions that are valuable in building a helping dialogue. The two that I intend briefly to focus on are questions and reflections. People suffering serious psychiatric disorders may often experience what Perkins and Repper (1996) refer to as 'cognitive overload'. It can be difficult for people to process and make sense of experience, which may be communicated to others in vague, confused, disconnected, distracted ways. Conversations that are too probing or intense can overload vulnerable people and lead to withdrawal, avoidance, or the exacerbation of acute symptoms. Others may be so sunk in depression they seem difficult to engage with. Others may be troubled and distracted by unusual thoughts or voice hearing. In all these scenarios sensitivity and awareness in the use of these skills is required.

It is usually more appropriate and helpful to ask open questions (see assessment guide below). The client is better able to communicate how they experience their problems and needs and do not feel intimidated by a string of closed questions which are often related to the practitioner's agenda and perception of the presenting problems. Follow-up questions can be used to focus down on specific issues. They may be concerned with getting clarity – 'You seem to be saying that facing the day seems so difficult that you give up. Is that how it is?' They may be used to encourage people to say more – 'So you say you that in the past when you felt bad you coped better. How did you do that?' Follow-up questions can be used to encourage the client to reconsider some aspect of their experience – 'You say you used to enjoy things but you can't now. How do you know?' A further way in which follow-up questions are commonly used is to identify the relevance of something that's said – 'You said earlier that people never listen, never take you seriously. I'm wondering if you feel you have to threaten to do something worrying before anyone will listen?' Probes may also be non-verbal, as when we use an expression or gesture to encourage someone to say more, or they can also take the form of minimal verbal prompts. We need to be aware that there is often concern in the minds of people about how what they confide will be seen. 'Will they think I'm mad, bad or stupid? Will they understand? Will they dislike and disapprove of me? Will they put me in hospital?'

There are a number of disadvantages related to a conversational style that relies too heavily on asking questions. First, it tends to locate the power with the practitioner – she decides what is talked about and directs the conversation. Second, there is a danger that questions can be asked in a routine unthinking manner and are not responsive to the uniqueness of an individual's experience. A further disadvantage is that people will only reply to what is asked and significant areas of the client's experience are not discussed.

It is good practice to develop the ability to respond reflectively in our dialogues with people in care. Reflections involve restating or mirroring back what the client has disclosed of their experience. They involve feeding back what we have heard and understood of what the client has said – the content, and the affective element. We should take care that we are restating in our own words what the client has said and not constructing a reality that does not match the client's experience. Discerning the more subtle or suppressed emotional experience of the client can be difficult and the reflection of feeling is best expressed in a tentative way. Used skilfully, reflective responses can communicate a high degree of empathy, identified by Carl Rogers (Mearns and Thorne, 1999) as a core therapeutic condition.

Being reflective creates a dialogue in which the practitioner is not setting the agenda and directing the flow of the conversation. There is a shared responsibility for what gets talked about. Hargie *et al.* (1994), in a review of the research on reflective interviews, conclude that they are more likely to result in the development of more positive attitudes towards the practitioner and an increase in the amount and intimacy of the disclosures.

A silence that occurs in conversations between the practitioner and client can be disconcerting for both but it is more acceptable and tolerable where a comfortable, safe relationship has been established. We often feel a need to fill the silence, to say something, anything, to reduce the social anxiety we experience. Silence can have a particular quality. It can be a resentful or angry silence; an anxious distracted silence; a reflective thoughtful silence; an uncertain reticent silence; an evasive guarded silence; a deep despairing silence; an estranged isolated silence; or a submissive deferring silence. It is important to develop sufficient comfort with silences to allow them and assess their meaning. Profound feelings can be expressed in this way. Acceptance of the silence needs to be communicated through relaxed attentive body language. Sometimes being quiet with someone who has little energy to talk, or is too distracted by anxiety, or who needs the recuperative sanctuary of silence, can be experienced as extremely supportive. Responding sensitively to silence can lead to important issues, concerns and feelings being shared and discussed. The way we respond will depend on how we assess the silence. For example – 'It seems difficult to continue, almost too painful to talk about;' 'My guess is that in your silence you are saying you feel pretty resentful about being here', or simply 'What's on your mind?' – may be appropriate.

Assessment guide

The following guide is offered as a way of bringing some structure to your assessment interviews and conversations with clients. You may need to rephrase the questions to fit with your conversational style. The structure is holistic and aims to engage clients in an exploratory conversation about the physical, psychological, social and spiritual dimensions of their world in a way that throws some light on their distress, the problems of living they face and the needs they have. Some of the questions can be quite challenging and should always be asked in a respectful and supportive way. The questions are orientated towards the past, present and future. A frequent criticism of psychiatric interviewing is that it is often 'archaeological', with too much focus on digging up and exploring the past and not enough focus on the challenges of the here and now and pathways towards a preferred future. While insight into 'the past in the present' may be an ingredient in change for some people, for others it offers no solution to their present distress and no solution to their search for a different way of being in the world. Egan argues that from an early point in our engagement with people we should be looking towards possibilities for change and seeking strategies to bring this about. Often people are already making tentative moves in the direction of desired change, or making use of positive coping strategies to manage their distress, although not perhaps fully exploiting them. Bringing this future orientation and solution focus to the conversation instils a sense of hope. Some examples of future and solution orientated questions are included in the sections 'Creating a Better Future' and 'Creating Strategies to Move Forward' in Part 2.

Another criticism is that nursing assessments tend to have a medical/symptom orientation or that they tend to be to problem focused. As I have suggested elsewhere, despite the challenge of person-centred and other psycho-social perspectives on human distress, the biomedical model remains dominant in psychiatric practice and also significantly influences nursing practice. Nurses then approach assessment from a diagnostic perspective and are principally concerned with identifying the symptoms of, for example, depression, or the positive and negative symptoms of schizophrenia. Nursing assessments and the assessments of other mental health professionals often become a ritual in which the person's problem-saturated story is retold. What White (1997) calls a 'thin' narrative of a person's lived experience becomes the defining story. The more often it is told, the more the person comes to see himself as a problematic person, living a problematic life.

Nursing assessment should not be symptom focused or problem orientated, although we might engage clients in conversations about those aspects of their experience. Instead, it should be person orientated and concerned with understanding their way of being in the world and how that might change in ways that would lead to less suffering. White talks about the need for conversations that bring out the full richness of an individual's lived experiences, not the edited problem-laden versions. This is where assessment and recovery become interwoven in the helping process. As we engage clients in 'thicker' narratives, or other stories of their lived experience, in which their qualities, talents, strengths, achievements and resources are visible, when nurturing, life-enhancing events occurred, a different identity can begin to emerge.

I do not much care for the term assessment. It symbolizes for me the power differential in helping relationships, where one person who has the expertise and knowledge assesses a client who has limited or no knowledge of what their distress means and little expertise to help themselves. Setting out the structure as a series of questions gives the impression of an interview in which the agenda is set by the practitioner. I visualize it much more as a collaborative dialogue in which the client's story unfolds and is filled out in the context of a developing relationship. Often very few questions need to be asked if nurses can create a secure base from which the 'territory of distress' can be explored. If we can be an empathic presence, accept a person's reality without trying too hard try to explain it, people will return from the territory of their distress having learnt something about themselves and will have begun the process of recovery. It is when experience is explained away according to this dogma or that, that the seeker of truth about themselves and their lives surrenders to passive resignation and the spirit of recovery fades.

An overview of the problem

'Can you say a little about what's been happening to you?'
'What do you feel you need help with?'
'Can you say a little about how you see the problem?'
'What things have been troubling you?'
'How is it affecting you/others?'

'How bad is it? On a scale of 1–10, where 10 is the worst it's ever been, where are you today?'

'How have you been coping? What has helped?'

How has your behaviour changed?

'What's become difficult for you?'

'What would you like to be able to do that you don't do now?'

'What happens when you begin to get depressed/high? What do you first notice? What else?'

'How do you know when you're becoming unwell/becoming troubled again?' 'What do you first notice?'

'What changes have other people noticed in you?'

'What do you notice yourself doing more of the time?'

'Do you find yourself avoiding people/places?'

'Have you noticed any change in your level of interest in things?'

'Do you find yourself doing things because your voices tell you to?'

'Is your behaviour more worrying for you or for others?'

'On a scale of 1–10, where 10 is that you will do anything to overcome this problem and 1 is there's nothing you can do but hope, where would you put yourself?'

Do you ever have thoughts of harming yourself/killing yourself? How often/how detailed/how persistent?'

'What's stopped you acting on these thoughts?'

'Do you ever have thoughts of harming others? How often/how detailed/how persistent?'

'What's stopped you acting on these thoughts?'

'On a scale of 1–10, how worried should I be about you harming yourself/killing yourself/harming others, over the next week?'

The response to this last series of questions may indicate a need for a further and more detailed risk assessment.

How has your mood changed?

'How have you been feeling?'

'Can you describe the feeling for me?'

'Do you find yourself getting upset easily?'

'Are there times when you feel better?'

'How bad is your anxiety/depression at the moment? On a scale of 1–10, with 10 being the worst, where are you today?'

'How are you managing to cope when it's so bad?'

'What helps when you feel like this?'

'What happens to your anger/ sadness/fearfulness?'

'Where in your body do you experience it?'

How have you been affected mentally?

'What concerns you most? What's your worst fear?'

'When you are depressed/anxious in those situations, what are your thoughts?'

'How is your concentration/memory/speed of thought?'

'Do you have thoughts that trouble you?'

'How did you come to believe that? What was happening in your life around the time you first began to think that?'

'What leads you believe that? What evidence do you have that's what's happening?'

'How sure are you that what you believe to be happening is true? On a scale of 1–100, with 100 being absolute conviction, where would you put yourself?'

'Has anything happened recently that's increased/decreased your conviction?'

'How persistent are these thoughts? Do you find yourself thinking about it most of the time/some of the time/occasionally?'

'How are you affected by these thoughts? How do you feel/react when you get these thoughts?'

'Do you ever have the experience of voices talking to you that others can't hear?'

'What do theses voices sound like/what do they say/when do you notice them most/how do they affect you/can you resist them?'

'How do you explain them?'

'How do you react to them?'

How have you been affected physically?

'How do you feel physically?'

'Have you had any physical problems lately? What do you attribute that to?'

'How do you take care of your body?'

'How do you feel about your body?'

'How's your energy?'

'How have you been sleeping? If there were a reason for you to stay awake, what do you think that would be?'

'What dreams have you remembered recently? If that dream had a title, what would it be? What connections do you make with that image in your dream? What feelings were around in the dream? What part of your life do those feelings belong to?'

'How have you been eating?'

'Do you experience any pain/discomfort in any part of you body?'

'When do you experience that? How bad is it on a scale of 1–100?'

'How do you cope with it? What helps? How do others react?'

'If your pain/discomfort was telling you something, what do you think that might be?'

'Allow your attention to focus on the part of your body that experiences pain/discomfort for a few minutes. What images/thoughts come to mind?'

'Do you have any worries about your sexual relationship. What concerns do you have about your sexual life?'

'Have you been using any recreational drugs lately?'

'In what ways have your prescribed drugs helped? Are you experiencing any troublesome side effects?'

How have you been affected socially?

'How are your relationships with your partner/children/parents?'
'Have there been any changes in your family relationships/friendships recently?'
'How have your family relationships/friendships been affected?'
'What relationships are important in your life? How are these?'
'What's good about your life at the moment?'
'What's missing from your life at the moment?'
'What areas of your life need attention/need to change?'
'How do you spend your time/your day?'
'What gives you pleasure/what interests you?'
'How are you managing at work? How is not having a job affecting you?'
'Do you notice any change in the way people are with you?'
'How has your life been affected by having this mental health problem?'
'What's the one single change that would make most difference to your life right now?'
'Who or what makes life difficult for you?'
'How do you feel about talking with someone of the opposite sex/a different sexual orientation/ethnic background?'
'Could you say something about your culture that would help me understand a little more about you?'
'Have you experienced discrimination/prejudice? How has that affected you?'
'What does home mean to you? Do you have that at this point in your life?'

What sort of stresses have you been under recently?

'What changes have taken place in your life recently?'
'What's been difficult in your life lately?'
'What things are a worry at home/work/school?'
'If you could change something in your life right now, what would it be?'
'What was happening in your life when you first began to have problems?'

Does this connect with your family background/personal history?

'Could you say a little about your background – whatever comes to mind?'
'Could you tell me a little about your/father/mother/siblings?'
'Could you tell me a little about your early life?'
'Could you say a little about school/college?'
'Who were the other important figures in your life? Who were your mentors/models as you were growing up?'
'Can you scan back to times when you've felt this way before?'
'If you the child were sitting on that chair now, what would you want to say to him/her?'
'If your father/mother were sitting here right now, what would you want to say?

What in your life do you find inspiring/dispiriting?

'Does your faith play a important part in your life?'
'Is prayer/contemplation/meditation important in your life?'
'What are the things in your life that give it meaning?'
'What sort of experiences have brought you a sense of joy/peace to your life?'
'Are there some things in life that lift you out of the everyday business of living and into a more exalted state of mind?'
'Are there some virtues that are important to you in the way you live your life? How difficult is it to live up to those ethical standards? How are you affected when you don't?'
'Where do you go/what do you do when you want to find a sense of peacefulness?'
'What are some of the things that have happened in your life that have given you a feeling of goodness/when you've experienced a sense of goodness in others?'

What sort of help do you think you need?

'When you've felt like this before, what has helped you most? What else?'
'How has that helped'?
'How do you think I/we could help? How would that help?'
'What would help you most at the moment?'
'What makes it easier for you to cope?'
'Is there anything you can do to help yourself get through this?'
'What is the thing that is most difficult/worrying/distressing/urgent that you would like help with right now?'
'Is there one thing that it would possibly be helpful to work on right now?'

Could you say a little about the good things in your life, the things that are OK?

'What are the things in your life that you get pleasure/satisfaction from?'
'What are some of the things you enjoy/are interested in?'
'What are you good at? What would the person who knows you best say you were good at?'
'What are some of the things that you've done that you are proud of/get a sense of satisfaction from?'
'Who are the people that are important in your life?'
'Who do you turn to if you need help?'
'Have there been times when other people have had to rely on you/when you've helped others out?'
'Tell me about a time in your life when you felt happy/secure?'
'What's the best job you've ever had/what sort of work would you like to do?'
'How do you look after yourself/stay well?'
'How do you relax?'
'What's kept you going through all the difficult times?'

'When things have been difficult for you, what do you do/what do other people do that helps?'

'What are some of your hopes for the future?'

'If you had overcome these problems, what would your life look like/how would your life be different?'

'If I had met you a few years back, what would I have noticed about you that's different from how you are now?'

'If I was talking to someone who knows you really well/knows all your best qualities/good points, what would they tell me?'

Self-enquiry Box

As a general principle we should not ask other people questions we are not prepared to ask ourselves! You may find it interesting to consider the question, 'Which area of my life needs most attention right now?' Select some relevant questions from the assessment framework (or frame your own) and respond to them.

You may find it useful to use a free associative writing technique in which you allow your answer to emerge in what you write. Try not to deliberate and evaluate, just write. Don't worry about spelling or grammar. Just keep your pen moving and write whatever comes into your mind.

5 Creating pathways to recovery

Come to the edge
He said. They said:
We are afraid.
Come to the edge
He said. They came.
He pushed them and they flew.

Guillaume Apollinaire (source unknown).

Recovery is the process of becoming a fully functioning person and reclaiming life. It is a deeply personal experience that involves changing one's attitudes, values and feelings, goals, skills and roles. It is a pathway towards a satisfying, hopeful and contributing life despite (or perhaps because of) the limitations caused by enduring mental health problems (see Figure 5.1). Recovery involves the development of new meaning and purpose in one's life as one grows beyond the catastrophic effects of mental illness. On the whole, mental health services have created a culture of maintenance rather than recovery, in which people with severe mental health problems can become trapped in a career as a mental patient. An attitude of therapeutic pessimism has developed in relation to working with deeply troubled people. There is an expectation of relapse and increasing disability, a belief that the best one can hope for is symptom control. The missing ingredient in so many care and treatment programmes is hope and a belief in the potential of people to change and grow, to become more resourceful human beings and engage more fully in life. In a culture of maintenance, people are offered supportive services, but have little opportunity to engage in a recovery programme which is enabling and which nurtures their growth as a person. What needs to be recognized is that people are disabled not so much by their vulnerabilities as by the anguish, despair and hopelessness that builds up around it (Deegan, 1988).

People who are in recovery often talk of significant turning points that changed the direction of their lives from breakdown and disintegration, to breakthrough and reintegration. This often seems to involve the presence of another person who is able to relate to them in a way that is enabling. As Deegan puts it, 'It is the loving invitation to be something more' (p. 14). In a similar vein, Rogers (1977) describes a humanistic alternative to the biomedical approach and conventional care. He suggests that deeply troubled

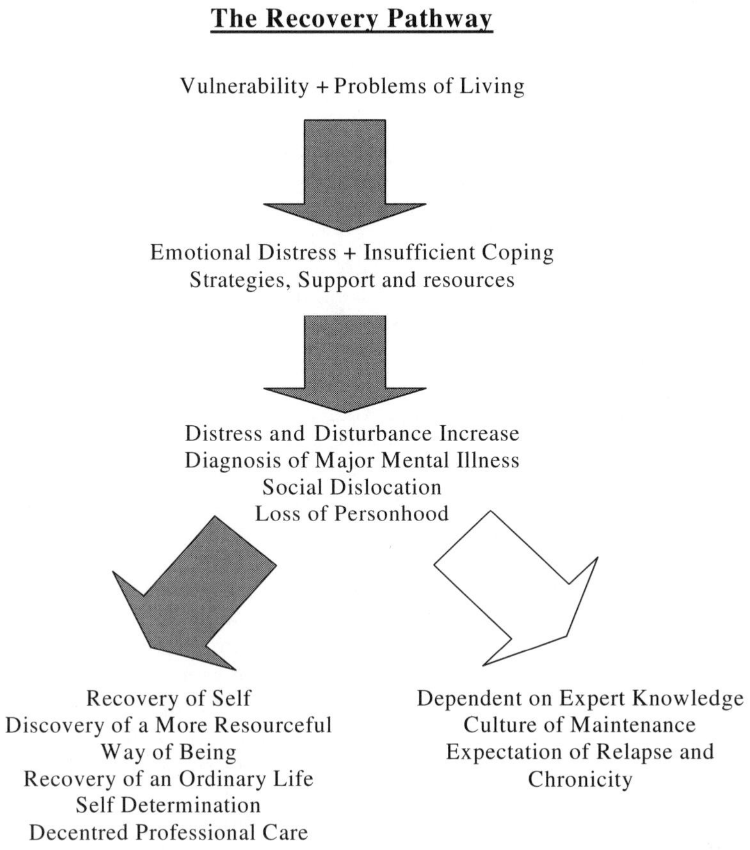

The Recovery Pathway

Vulnerability + Problems of Living

Emotional Distress + Insufficient Coping
Strategies, Support and resources

Distress and Disturbance Increase
Diagnosis of Major Mental Illness
Social Dislocation
Loss of Personhood

Recovery of Self
Discovery of a More Resourceful
Way of Being
Recovery of an Ordinary Life
Self Determination
Decentred Professional Care

Dependent on Expert Knowledge
Culture of Maintenance
Expectation of Relapse and
Chronicity

Figure 5.1 The recovery pathway

individuals who are expressing themselves in ways that are frequently described as psychotic, can be seen as going through a chaotic stressful period of growth and in need of understanding and companionship rather than interventions that emphasize directive care and suppression of symptoms.

Recovery is a process of learning about oneself, of discovering oneself. It is a unique journey that follows different paths. Podroll (1990) describes it as a journey that can require 'valiant personal action and a life-long commitment to health'. He argues that even in the midst of madness one can recognize the seeds of recovery, which he refers to as 'islands of clarity', in which the individual regains, albeit briefly, footholds in 'reality' and engages constructively in living. These moments grow as the journey of recovery begins. It is seldom a straightforward journey. Even people someway along the road can lose their psychological bearings, stumble and become lost again in a psychotic terrain. However, once people have begun their journey, these setbacks can be temporary and they are able to retrace their steps and regain the recovery pathway. Relapses while in recovery can be seen not as failures, but potential periods of growth, in which people are not so much breaking down as breaking through and moving forward. Matthew, a young man in recovery, with a long history of being overwhelmed by 'psychotic' experiences is an example of this. He again became disturbed and distressed by unusual thoughts and derogatory voices during a period when he was trying to establish himself on a horticulture course at a local college and required a brief period of 'time out' in respite accommodation that provided support and sanctuary. Rather than see this as a failure it was seen as a courageous effort by him to develop his talent, secure a socially valued role for himself and to rise to the challenge of relating to and finding acceptance in a group of peers. The supportive and inclusive response of his peers to his revealed vulnerability marked a breakthrough for Matthew. It allowed to him to experience himself as a valued, liked and respected person and strengthened his hope for a life as a full citizen rather than as a marginalized life of a person with a psychiatric disability.

We need to construct a therapeutic milieu in which relapses are seen as expected events in a person's journey of recovery and not further steps on a deteriorating course towards disability and dependency (White, 1987). They can be seen as episodes of 'time out' from the continuing struggle to claim an ordinary life. It can be helpful in recovery work to assist individuals to recognize their relapse signature (early signs) and to implement an agreed crisis plan, which may or may not include a brief admission to hospital or a short stay in some other appropriate sanctuary. A crisis episode can be used as an opportunity for learning that can enable people to regain a firmer foothold on the recovery path. Where there is a history of multiple admissions, White suggests that it can be useful to schedule a number of periods of time out during the year. These planned admissions are less demoralizing, more empowering than crisis admissions. They can be opportunities to acknowledge progress and recognize the demands that staying in recovery makes, particularly on those with limited social support systems. After the first series of scheduled admissions, it becomes possible for the individual to experiment with longer intervals between periods of time out. For some people it is having this locus of support as an option that is comforting and sustaining and paradoxically reduces the uptake.

Angie's story *(Theme: the recovery process)*
Angie is a young woman with a 10-year history of serious self-harm and frequent referrals to acute in patient services. She has a deeply negative self-concept and correspondingly low self-esteem, which she disguises behind a thin veneer of emotional buoyancy and outgoingness. Frequently escalating psychosomatic tension and bleak feelings about herself and her life break through to the surface and capsize her mood. It is at these times that she is gripped by an urge to cut or burn herself. Over the years the frequency and seriousness of her self-harming has increased, leading to an increase in the number and length of admissions. The admissions were demoralizing for Angie and seemed to be taking her in a

direction away from the 'ordinary life' which she craves. It is also demoralizing for the staff who began to see Angie as a 'chronic self-harmer' with a 'damaged manipulative personality', for whom very little could be done. They experienced feelings of helplessness, guilt, anger, anxiety, distrust, sadness and perplexity in the face of Angie's continued self-mutilation.

The hypothesis about the nature of self-harming that seemed to fit for Angie was that injuring herself was both a solution and a problem. It was a solution in the sense that it had evolved as a way of externalizing her inner distress and of making visible a deep sense of hurt and betrayal that had been present from her childhood onwards, connected with her mother's abandonment of her and her father when she was four. Secondly, the physical pain gave her some sense of relief by displacing emotional pain in her conscious awareness. It was a problem in the obvious sense that her self-harming had become at times life threatening. It had also caused multiple disfiguring scars, which Angie was increasingly sensitive about and had made relationships and a working life impossible. The increasing frequency and severity of her self-injuries suggested that it was no longer a solution to her underlying distress.

A decision was made to 'appoint' Angie the expert on her own life. With the help of her key worker she was asked to construct a plan for recovering herself and her life from the grip of the problem of self-harm. The aim of this strategy was first to try to dis-identify the person from the problem. This was necessary because Angie's story had become so problem-saturated that other aspects of herself and her life had been all but eclipsed. Secondly, there was a need to demonstrate a trust in her ability to tap into her innate wisdom for a change that would make a difference; a way of responding to her distress that was different to the entrenched self-harm pattern and would begin the process of healing; to encourage in her a sense that she could become an agent in her own recovery, which was not dependent on professional help for the right medication programme, the right psychotherapeutic intervention.

Angie's perspective

'At first it was a shock to realize that they were serious, that I was being expected to prescribe my own care. It didn't feel like they had given up on me or abandoned me, because there was a lot of encouragement and my key worker spent time with me and was accessible. It was a relief to know that they were not going to try to prevent me from cutting myself. They recognized that for me it was a way of coping with my feelings and until I had some other way of coping, there would still be times when I would need to self-harm. They were more concerned about me doing it safely with as less damage as possible. Strangely, the fact that I could do it seemed to lessen my need to do it and I soon found that I had gone five weeks without cutting, which is close to a record for me. Of course it didn't last. I think what was helpful in the first few months was the feeling, for the first time really, that I was being heard. Also not being treated like a 'bad girl' but respectfully, like an adult. I began to think maybe I could take better care of myself and not damage myself so much, maybe I'm worth it. That was on good days. At other times any good and hopeful feelings I had about myself were crushed by this feeling of desolation and the thought that there would never be anything good in my life, because there was nothing good in me. With my key worker I developed a schedule of strategies that I would work through if I felt like self-harming when I was at home in my flat:

- Do something active and vigorous (take a walk, dance, do some hand washing).
- Negotiate with myself to postpone self-harming for 12 hours.
- Look at my therapeutic documents.
- Telephone my key worker/ support worker or the crisis line.
- Paint or draw vigorously using finger paints or charcoal.
- Take an aromatherapy bath.
- Listen to guided imagery tape.
- If I need to cut, use a clean guarded blade to limit the extent of the injury.
- Take responsibility for dressing cuts and getting myself to A&E if I need stitches.

In addition, I had an agreement that if I was feeling overwhelmed and couldn't cope without cutting I could go into hospital for a day or two.

As well as seeing my key worker twice a week I joined an art therapy group and attended a support group for women who self-harm. My self-harm rate has now gone down from about five times a month to one in the last three months. I'm feeling a whole lot stronger emotionally and more positive about myself. I had lost sight of so many things in my life history that affirmed a different identity from the hateful person that I'd become. It's been a bit like editing a story so that the life of the central character is not so swamped by misfortune that their life can only be seen as a tragedy and end tragically.

Early steps in an individual's recovery are tentative. People can feel extremely vulnerable as they encounter their emerging selves and begin to reclaim their lives. Demoralization and disempowerment are commonly experienced and are significant barriers to recovery. It is important that these early steps are manageable and achievable and that people do not go too far out on a limb before the limb has grown strong enough to support them. Each small step needs to be acknowledged as evidence of an underlying healing process at work and can be worked with to encourage hopefulness and self-direction and to rebuild self-esteem and confidence. Out of these therapeutic moments come turning points. For some it might be having their subjective reality understood deeply and empathically by another person that draws them back into the world. For others it might be daring to believe that a different life is possible or, alternatively, the experience of an accomplishment that awakens a sense of personal agency.

Fisher (1999) emphasizes the importance of reoccupying a valued social role as a key factor in recovery. Re-establishing oneself in the world of work, becoming a student or becoming a tenant and neighbour are examples of this. Maintaining one's place within a family and a community that provides an emotional ambience conducive to recovery. In short, retaining (or regaining) one's social integration and citizenship are important to recovery and continued well-being. Evidence for this has come from the World Health Organisation's (WHO) comparative studies on the course and outcome of severe mental disorder in a number of countries that span the spectrum of socioeconomic development. That the outcome is significantly better in developing countries which use fewer drugs and less hospitalization, challenges the view that a highly professionalized care system is the best guarantee for improving the long-term course of schizophrenia (de Girolamo, 1996).

What seems to become clear through what many people say about their 'breakthroughs' and 'turning points' is the importance of autonomy and connectedness. It is when people begin to become self-determining and take responsibility for themselves and their lives that change begins. Until that step is taken, life is lived according to the conditions of others, often in the context of controlling, dependent relationships, with all the limitations that that imposes and people will not experience themselves as agents in their own healing process. Lives are rebuilt on hope, a willingness to act and responsible action (Deegan, 1988). The legacy of disability from the era of institutional psychiatry and from patterns of care in the community that replicate an institutional model, should be sufficient evidence of the damage that segregated care can do. When we become disconnected from the social moorings that anchor us in the broad stream of a shared reality and the norms and values of our culture, we are set adrift in a sea of madness. The WHO studies should alert us to the possibility that chronicity is not the natural outcome of severe mental disorder but what Illich (1977) has called the iatrogenic outcome of psychiatric treatment and care.

Ben's story *(Theme: the recovery process)*
It's about 5 years since I last had to go into hospital. I still see my CPN once a month, more frequently if I'm getting too high or too low. We've got to know each other pretty well over the years so our conversations are not all about my hassles, they are about what's going on for her as well. I feel much more comfortable with that. Before, I often used to feel like I was an observed object, part of some global experiment in mind control. I was having to take a lot of prescribed drugs at that time and I suppose I would be what people call a non-compliant patient. Only to my mind I wasn't

being non-compliant, I was adopting life-saving tactics. Discovering my diagnosis was a devastating experience. My first encounter with my diagnosis was seeing paranoid schizophrenic written on my case notes; it was literally soul destroying. Recently I've written to a psychiatrist asking if I can have that diagnosis rescinded. I hate the idea of being tagged for life. Now, apart from Cathy my CPN, I have no other contact with the psychiatric services and only take medication when I need to.

Things began to change when I saw a new psychiatrist who actually listened to me and I began to feel I had some control over my life. He encouraged me to write down what I was experiencing and discuss it with him if I wanted to. I had learnt in my career as a psychiatric case that you didn't say much to the doctors or nurses because they would simply write you up as disturbed, give you more medication and keep you in hospital. For me writing was the breakthrough. At first I just wrote narrative, 'A day in the death of Benjamin Salthouse', that sort of thing. But then I found that I could write prose poems. I'd never read any poetry before but I'd always had an ear for the lyrics of the music I was into at that time. When I look back at some of those early poems, a lot of them were about a young black guy who had no sense of identity. Even my self-image had walked out on me. I was in need of an image consultant, not a psychiatrist. One of the voices I heard during that time was a black angel. She used to tell me I was 'one step away from God'. I found it both comforting and alarming. When I was low I used to think I was about to die a violent death at the hands of a friendly assassin. Often I thought that the nurses were trying to kill me. When I was high, I used to think I was in some way special, that I was chosen, that I was the black envoy of God.

A lot of people encouraged me. At some level I was able to see myself held together in the ordered structure and rhythm of the poems. My chaotic, unreal world seemed no more than an awakened dream that had escaped from the night. This was narcosis, not psychosis. Who I am now struggled into existence in the poems and waited for me to catch up. For me writing is therapy. There are still times when my reality becomes confusing and I get overwhelmed and may behave in unwise ways. But I'm much better at recognizing that these days. I know that what I need to do is to find a quiet retreat somewhere, where I can take respite from the world for a few weeks.

In the process of recovery, chemotherapy and psychotherapy can be seen as self-determined strategies the individual recognizes as being a part of their holistic self-care. But we should guard against giving any therapy the status of a panacea. For recovering and sustaining our well-being we all need to build into our lives experiences which are nourishing, strengthening and healing. An inspiring example of this is Rene whose life was for many years disrupted and all but destroyed by her immobilizing lows and chaotic highs.

Rene's story *(Theme: the recovery process)*
Rene is a 37-year-old woman with a history of manic depressive disorder dating back to her early 20s. A precipitating event seemed to be the sudden death of her father who sexually abused her until her early teens. This had remained a secret in the family until his death. Over the next few years Rene was admitted to hospital several times. She attempted suicide on two separate occasions and was drinking heavily. Medication seemed to help when she became depressed or manic, but was ineffective in stabilizing her mood. Rene, with the help of her CPN, was able to identify the early signs of her deepening lows or escalating highs and become familiar with her relapse signature. Together they were able to construct a recovery plan that she could use to balance her mood. Making adjustments to her self-medication programme was just one strategy in a plan that involved switching to a quieter lifestyle when the early signs of a high were recognized and engaging in a manageable and nurturing activity schedule when she recognized a significant down-swing. She also had some alcohol counselling and later some psychotherapy. This enabled her to let go of an image of herself as a flawed and worthless human being whom other people found unappealing. Instead, she began to develop a more respectful attitude towards herself and to discover the 'treasure' hidden within her unfolding self. Some pastoral counselling from a chaplain helped Rene rediscover the comfort and inspiration of prayer and contemplation and helped fill a spiritual emptiness that enveloped her life with meaninglessness. All of this took courage and a willingness to invest energy in discovering herself and recovering her life. It was not straightforward. There were many doubts and setbacks along the way. Perhaps a key factor was the co-creation of motivation. We tend to see motivation as goal-directed energy that comes from within. But often motivation is the product of the social system or interpersonal context of which the individual is part. In Rene's case her sustained motivation came out of a respectful, encouraging, enabling therapeutic system; a system that involved her family, her key worker, a psychiatrist and other professional mental health workers whom she chose to work with at various points in her recovery.

Recovery involves giving our attention to the four dimensions of human experience: body, mind, spirit and our social world. A sense of well-being is derived from achieving a degree of balance and harmony within and between our internal and external worlds. Achieving this balance has traditionally been an integral part of the healing process in Eastern cultures. In the West, we persist in seeing problems associated with the way we feel, think and behave as illness. This way of conceptualizing distress is alien to people from many African and Asian cultures and, it should be said, alien to a growing number of people in the West (Fernando, 1995). Historically, in Western psychiatry and psychotherapy the mind and body have been split, the social context of distress ignored and the spirit neglected.

People in recovery are reclaiming sovereignty over their lives. They are defining for themselves the meaning of their distress and making choices and decisions about what will help in their recovery. People now think of themselves as consumers of the mental health services, as members of rehabilitation or resource centres and in the context of oppressive social and psychiatric systems as survivors. However, Deegan (1997) advises caution in thinking that new labels necessarily reflect a change in the relationship between those labelled and those not labelled. People who have experienced serious mental health problems still find a significant power difference and a lack of mutuality in their relationships with professional helpers. White (1997) describes an approach to professionalized helping, which he calls de-centred care, in which a consciousness of the power difference enables helpers to stay mindful of potential abuses. Maintaining this awareness opens up the possibility of exploring the way in which other relations of power have influenced the construction of people's stories and identity. The way in which the abuse, injustice and oppression that exists in our culture in everyday interactions, is reflected in the stories people hold and tell about their lives. In de-centred care the therapeutic endeavour places the client's knowledge of their lived experience at the centre of the work, rather than the professional's 'expert' knowledge. White's contention is that the therapeutic encounter should provide a context in which the stories of people's lived experience are told, both the known and the 'missing' narratives. It is in that telling and re-telling that detail emerges of alternative story lines to the dominant problem-laden story that is replayed again and again in the conventional psychiatric interview. In the re-telling we discover courageous struggles against oppression and disadvantage. We find acts of care and kindness towards others. We find demonstrations of responsibility and wise action. We find accounts of relationships in which the client has been the object of loving attention. The re-authoring of lives in the light of these recovered stories nurtures the growth of a different stronger identity from the negative and limiting self-concept that exists in many people who are deeply troubled. As White puts it, the re-plotting of dominant narratives and the telling of previously untold stories become 'expressions of persistence, determination, struggle, protest, resistance and connectedness that come to represent a turning point in a person's life'.

Staff attitudes are very important in creating a culture of recovery. There is an illusory belief among many mental health professionals that somehow they are able rise above the anguish and struggle of human existence. As professional helpers, we need to be aware of our own wounds and to live the spirit of recovery in our own lives. The dynamic healing environment is one in which staff members are vitally involved in their own growth and recovery. As Deegan suggests, it is this that allows us to empathize deeply with the wounds and vulnerability of people in our care. Real community is not a place, it is an inclusive attitude based on the recognition of a shared humanity.

White uses the phrase 'taking it back' to describe the reciprocal nature of therapeutic relationships. He argues that in de-centred practice the therapeutic encounter can be nurturing and sustaining to the helper in a number of ways. In examining the way power is held and used in the helping relationship and in the wider social context, we are challenged to reflect on our own experience of power, both in the professional and personal sphere of our lives. Acknowledging the act of trust that is involved in allowing the helper into the person's life prompts into awareness the meaning of being included (or excluded) for the helper and their lives. Joining with people in the recovery of stories that lead to a change in identity and life direction can awaken the professional helper to what is being overlooked in their own lives, to neglected experience that provides a richer narrative account of their life journey and reshapes their identity. Similarly, listening to stories of the relational experience of client's lives can reconnect the helper with figures in their own histories. The reliving and revising of these narratives can increase our knowledge of our lived experience in a way that is healing. Being with people, witnessing their aspirations and actions in their journey towards a preferred way of being can cause ripples in the helper's own life. The stories clients tell are often graphic metaphors of the struggles of the human spirit to triumph over adversity. These storied images are carried into the helper's work and life in a sustaining way. Both in humanistic and narrative approaches to helping, the knowledge on which solutions to the problems of living are based are generated by the person seeking help. This 'solution knowledge' and the style of therapeutic conversations in which it is drawn out are learnt from the client and carried by the helper into subsequent work with others. In these and in other ways the helper is both giver and receiver in the therapeutic encounter.

Assumptions of a recovery-orientated service

- Recovery can take place without professional intervention. Professionals do not hold the key to recovery. People's own resources – their coping strategies, family and social support system – may be equally important. The task of professionals is to facilitate the recovery process.
- A common denominator of recovery is the presence of people who believe in and stand by the individual on their journey. If professionals cannot believe in the person, they can hinder the recovery process.
- A recovery vision does not require a particular view of an individual's vulnerability to disabling distress. Whether vulnerability and disability are viewed as primarily biological, psychosocial or spiritual, recovery is still a necessary process.
- Recovery can occur even though symptoms of distress remain and recur. Recovery is about living a valued and valuable life with difficulties, not alleviating them altogether.
- Recovery means that distress symptoms interfere less with a person's ability to live an ordinary life. They are less of a barrier to the expression and development of skills, talents, interests, aspirations, relationships and citizenship. A person is able to manage their problems more effectively.
- Recovery is not a linear process. It involves periods of personal growth and setbacks. Grieving for what has been lost as a consequence of an enduring vulnerability to disabling distress is part of the recovery process.
- Recovery from the social consequences of mental health problems can be more difficult than recovering from the disabilities themselves. The stigma, discrimination and disadvantage that people with enduring mental health problems experience can be a huge barrier to life as a full citizen.
- Recovery is a process of transcending an enduring vulnerability to disabling, distress. It requires hopefulness, courage, resolve, motivation and resourcefulness. These qualities are more likely to emerge and be sustained in the context of compassionate relationships with professional helpers and others.

Source: SW London and St Georges Mental Health Trust

6 A humanistic approach to helping

The humanistic approach to effective helping relationships can be summed up in the following beliefs:

- People are OK (though they might need help recognizing it).
- People can discover their own meanings (though they might need help doing it).
- People know what they need (though they might need help expressing it).
- People can take responsibility for themselves (though they might need encouragement to take it).

People are OK

A fundamental belief of the humanistic approach to helping is that every person is an individual of worth. Terms such as acceptance, respect and unconditional positive regard are widely used to describe the expression of this belief in the process of helping. Self-esteem is a major element in our sense of well-being. An inner core of positive self-regard enables us to enter life more confidently and express more of our potential. It helps protect us from the losses, failures, disappointments and rejections that are an inevitable part of life and threaten our self-concept. Without this inner core our self-esteem would be too externally regulated and overly vulnerable to adversity. A lack or loss of self-esteem is a problem facing many people who seek help from the mental health services. It can lie at the centre of the distress and the problems people face in living. Part of the experience of depression is an assault on a despised self, cognitively in the form of punishing and disabling self-talk and physically in the form of self-harm and suicidal behaviour. Others, particularly those with long-term or recurrent mental health problems, lose self-esteem as a consequence of becoming a patient. It can be demoralizing and undermining to face the stigma, social exclusion and disadvantage that people with mental health problems regularly encounter. Professionalized helping, too, can add to the diminution of self-esteem, by not involving people as agents in their own care and recovery process and by focusing too much on disabilities and vulnerabilities and not enough on talents, abilities and strengths (Chadwick, 1997). Building and strengthening self-esteem are important tasks in the recovery process. This can take place in context of a helping relationship in which the helper relates to the person in care in an authentic, accepting way. People need to feel valued and validated as a person. They need to feel that as they struggle to be themselves more fully they will not be judged or rejected. Acceptance must not be conditional on the individual being compliant and passively following advice and direction in order to retain the positive regard of the helper. Deegan (1992) argues that the very opposite of this, non-compliance and the assertion of autonomy, is necessary to the process of recovery. It is sometimes not easy for people to be open and receptive to the warmth and appreciation of others, so deeply embedded is their low self-esteem. They feel bad, hopeless, useless, unlovable as a person and this can only be resolved by re-evaluating the reasonableness of their negative self-concept in the light of a living learning experience that provides exceptions to that experience of themselves.

A belief in the essential worth of human beings is not to deny that we have a shadow side and that people sometimes behave in hurtful, damaging or evil ways. Humanistic thinking has in the past been criticized for having an overly optimistic view of human nature. The shadow side of human potential contains both negative destructive and positive constructive parts of ourselves that we are unable to own, largely as the result of the conditional love we have experienced during our development. We soon learn that to be acceptable and lovable certain behaviours are prohibited. The child whose playful exuberance is disapproved of may lose touch with their capacity to be enthusiastic, spontaneous and playful. If our distress and comfort-seeking behaviour is ignored, we may deny our emotional hurts and the need for comfort and support and express our distress in more damaging ways.

If our potential to be hateful, lustful, jealous, selfish, oppressive, remains an unacknowledged and unaccepted part of ourselves, there are likely to be a number of consequences. First, we use up a lot of energy repressing these aspects of ourselves, energy that is no longer available for living. Second, the more they are denied, the more likely they are to find expression in destructive projections, introjections and impulsive unwise acts. Third, the opposites of those traits are likely to be shallow representations of the real thing, a defensive reaction to the duality of self, captured in the colloquial saying, 'He's too good to be true'. The acknowledgement and acceptance of these potentials as part of our emergent self does not lead to them being expressed unrestrainedly. In fact the very opposite occurs. If we have autonomous choice, then we also have moral responsibility. Humanistic philosophy would argue that our choice is most often to move in the direction of constructive, wise action. Carl Rogers (Thorne, 1992) held the view that when we are in touch with our true self, then we have an inner sense of the rightness of our conduct in any given situation. He took the view that man was essentially a social being and that behaviour emanating from the true self would be socially constructive

It is difficult to reconcile this with the destructive behaviour of individuals, social groups and countries towards others. It sometimes seems as if the potential for antisocial behaviour and evil acts is in the ascendant at this moment in our history. There is then an even greater need at this moment in time for a philosophy that recognizes and liberates the human potential for love and compassion. There is a place within the context of humanistic philosophy for the spiritual and both Eastern and Western spiritual traditions have left their imprint on humanistic thinking. Thorne makes an interesting comparison between creation spirituality with its recognition of the divinity of all of nature and the hopeful view of human nature held by Rogers. To realize the divinity within us and around us nurtures a more reverential attitude towards ourselves, towards others and the world in which we live.

People can discover their own meanings

Since the late 19th century the biomedical model has dominated psychiatry. This pathologizing perspective on the experience of deeply troubled people not only depersonalizes and disempowers those seeking help, but also conflicts with humanistic nursing practice (Horsfall, 1997). At its most pernicious, pathologizing human experience is an invitation to infirmity. It legitimizes 'giving up the struggle' and enrols people in a 'career' as a psychiatric patient. Breggin (1996) takes up this theme, arguing that the biomedical model fails to value sufficiently the agency and personhood of service users. People can and need to be active forces in their own recovery. Approaches to helping deeply troubled people should respect, as much as possible, autonomy and freedom. At times it can seem as if the person has been all but eclipsed by the diagnostic label. The human qualities, talents and potentials the individual possesses have become submerged under the problem-saturated story (the psychiatric history). We are all authors. We all construct narratives of our lives and ourselves and use these stories to organize and give meaning to our experience. The stories we carry are selective narratives in the sense that they do not represent any absolute reality or capture what White and Epston (1990) call the full richness of any life experience. Our stories can be enabling and promote a sense of wellness or they can be undermining and disabling. In effect we become the central character in our stories as we re-enact them in our everyday lives. If our story is of being overwhelmed by life's challenges and the meaning drawn from that is that we are hopeless or inadequate or ill and unable to cope, we will become passive and helpless. If our dominant narrative is of failure and rejection, the meaning drawn from that might be that we are no good and we may express that in self-harm behaviour. The task of the helper is to facilitate a conversation in which people discover or co-create new meanings. The recovery process involves a shift, for example, from a person seeing themselves as bad to seeing themselves as more sinned against than sinning; from seeing themselves as a schizophrenic with a career as a psychiatric patient, to seeing themselves as a person with vulnerabilities (and abilities) that they can manage. This approach has its roots in social constructionism and the philosophy of Foucault. The central premise is that dominant social discourses can seem to objectify reality and lead to rigid inflexible perspectives on social experience against which we measure ourselves. These dominant social discourses, for example on gender, shape our personal narratives and influence, often in limiting and damaging ways, the way we see ourselves and live our lives.

In the context of biomedical psychiatry, the primary role of the nurse is to monitor people for symptom reduction in response to medication, for side effects of medication and for early signs of relapse. An extension of this role is the education of people in care and their families about medication and the biomedical construct of their presenting problems. This lends itself to a prescriptive, 'expert-led' approach to care and away from a partnership in care envisaged by recent reports on the future of mental health nursing (Department of Health, 1994). It presupposes that we know the cause (meaning) of a person's distressed and disturbed behaviour and know what they need in order to recover without necessarily asking them. The healing potential of the caring relationship is seen, if at all, as being peripheral to the client's recovery and leads to relationships becoming depersonalized and distant, a complaint frequently made in user satisfaction surveys. This contrasts starkly with humanistic nursing which emphasizes the therapeutic use of self, is empathetic to the experience of the person in care and seeks to work with them in egalitarian, empowering ways.

The dominance of the biomedical model has tended to minimize the social context as a significant factor in the client's experience of distress, disturbance and recovery. Schizophrenia is still predominantly seen as a physically based, pathological entity, despite the evidence for this view being strongly challenged by those who take a more psycho-social or psycho-spiritual perspective (Bentall, 1990; Boyle, 1990; Breggin, 1993). Depression is still primarily conceptualized as a disorder of neurotransmission despite the evidence that this common human experience of profound and debilitating despondency and despair is mediated by psychosocial factors (Brown, 1996). Humanistic philosophy, in emphasizing the whole being of the individual, the physical dimension, the psychological dimension, the spiritual dimension and the social dimension, as important components in the human experience of well-being, challenges the reductionist biomedical view of human suffering.

Humanistic approaches to helping are rooted in phenomenology. This is a method of enquiry employed in existential philosophy, which takes the view that knowledge and understanding can only be gained by exploring the subjective experience of people. Assumptions one holds about a phenomenon being explored are suspended and the researcher avoids imposing theoretical constructs on the experience of others. In the context of therapeutic helping the task is to enable others to report and describe their reality without interpreting it, without trying to fit it into some classification system. A shared explanatory hypothesis of what is going on and what is going wrong (and right as well) can evolve in a way that has meaningfulness for the client and is open to change in the light of further experience. Such an approach encourages trust and openness (Mosher and Burti, 1994). To call the experience of voice hearing an auditory hallucination and to interpret that as a symptom of a pathological syndrome called schizophrenia tells us very little about the nature and meaning of that experience to the individual. The work of Romme and Escher (1993) challenges the view that there is a causal connection between voice hearing and specific psychiatric disorders. They suggest that for many people voice hearing may be a survival strategy, a way of coping with trauma or some other adverse life situation, rather than a symptom of a particular disorder. Chadwick (1996) suggests that central to understanding psychotic phenomena is the human endeavour of trying to construct a sense of self that is valued and authentic. Events which are experienced as a threat to the sense of self, that trigger negative self-evaluation or lead to negative inferences about the intentions and evaluations of others, are common precipitants of disturbed, distressed behaviour. We need to work with people in ways that enable them to be open to and communicate their experience. It is the rediscovery or reconstruction of a sense of self that is a significant component in the recovery process in severe mental health problems (Davidson and Strauss, 1992).

Barker *et al.* (1997), in developing a construction of mental health nursing that is broadly humanistic, strike a note of opposition to what is seen as a reassertion of biomedical orthodoxy in psychiatric care. Mental health nursing is seen as primarily an interactive activity concerned with establishing the conditions necessary to promote the growth and development of the person in care. It is this emergent self and the personal resources this process releases that enables the person seeking help to manage the challenges of everyday living in less problematic ways. The focus of effective nursing is therefore seen as being person-centred rather than problem-centred. This process is seen as reflexive in the sense that it also influences the helper. I cannot be empathic with the experience of clients unless I am able to show myself that same empathy. As Deegan (1988) suggests, professional helpers need to acknowledge their own wounds and to live the spirit of recovery in their own lives. 'For professionals to accept and embrace their own woundedness and vulnerability is the first step towards understanding the experience of the disabled' (p. 18). Nursing is located in the context of the client's relational world: the client's relationship with self, with others, with the material world and with the spiritual. Nurses enter and, for a time, become part of the matrix of the whole, lived experience of the person in care.

People know what they need

The rhetoric in mental health care frequently extols the value of a needs-led service, i.e. a service that is responsive to the identified needs of the community. If this is not to remain empty rhetoric, the voice of user groups must be influential in determining service developments and priorities. A clear picture is emerging that significant numbers of people who use the services do not find the current provision helpful. There has been particular criticism of hospital-based acute services in meeting the needs of people in acute distress. In a recent study by service users, the three most important needs identified at times of acute distress were, someone to talk to; the need to feel safe and supported; and the need for somewhere to relax and calm down (Mental Health Foundation, 1997). These needs are unlikely to be met in an acute admission unit. As one respondent commented, 'When I have been ill, I have needed privacy and peace, neither of which I have had at all in hospital. I do need medication when I am in these states but I am convinced that the usual hospital environment is bad for me and when I am at my worst I am bad for other patients too'. A Sainsbury Centre survey also highlights the dissatisfaction of service users with acute services. This study concluded that 'hospital care is a non-therapeutic intervention' which often falls short of meeting the social and therapeutic needs of patients (Sainsbury Centre, 1998b). There are some hopeful signs of an emerging service that is responsive to the needs of people who become acutely disturbed and distressed. In some areas of the UK intensive community support is accessible to people 24 hours a day and sanctuaries (crisis houses) are available as an alternative to hospitalization. Studies show the effectiveness of these services, in a number of respects, to be as good as or an improvement on hospital care, while user satisfaction is higher (Minghella *et al.*, 1998).

It is not just acute services that fail to meet needs. Psychiatric care that is dominated by a cure-based approach or skills-based approach is unlikely to meet the needs of people with enduring mental health problems. The cure-based approach that identifies either psychopathology or neuropathology as problems to be fixed by a plethora of interventions, both medical and psychological, is of limited help to people who have ongoing vulnerabilities and increasing disabilities. Perkins and Repper (1996) argue that the cure-based approach can be positively damaging to both service users and staff because of the sense of demoralization and hopelessness that so often results when people do not recover or stay well. The cure-based approach can give rise to a culture of blame. Staff may feel they have failed and blame themselves, their colleagues, the system, or the patient and soon begin to suffer from burnout. Patients blame the staff or themselves and feel increasingly helpless and hopeless. Cure-based approaches have tended to overvalue 'the therapies' and undervalue care as a potent healing factor in the recovery process.

Skills-based approaches, which are widely used in psychiatric practice, tend to see people needs in terms of deficits. People may be assessed as lacking life skills or social skills and rehabilitation is seen as a process of increasing a person's competence in these areas. There are a number of problems with this. First, it can impose the values of professional helpers on to the person in care. A person may not value the ability to prepare a meal, preferring instead to use local cafés. They may not value independent living, which for them means social isolation, preferring instead the option of communal living. Second, it places the onus on the person with social disabilities to adapt to the community, whereas community acceptance of differentness would allow greater social inclusion. Would it be too much to expect a little more patience and tolerance towards a person whose inwardness and distraction made communicating with others in everyday life a little more tortuous than is usual? Finally, we should not confuse not using skills with not having skills. The former is far more common among mental health veterans and has more to do with demoralization than deficit. What is needed is not so much skills training as the presence of someone who can be with people in a way that is accepting and enabling. This is not a relationship that is overtly therapeutic. It does not demand anything of the person in care, it is a non-judgemental openness to wherever the person is, whether that be in a chaotic state of mind or in the first steps of recovery. Hallmarks of this relational style, which Mosher and Burti (1994) call 'letting be', are compassion, empathic understanding, validation, support and containment. There is a similarity between what is being described here as the art of being present and the Buddhist healing tradition of 'sending and taking'. Through meditation practice of sending out compassionate thoughts and taking in the anguish that is present in the world, practitioners train themselves to be with others in a way that allows them to resonate with deeply disturbed and distressed people and be with them in a way that is understanding, compassionate and restorative (Podroll, 1990). Being present with people can give way to a more active involvement and collaborative problem solving as their psychosocial needs become known as they begin to re-engage in life. The essential element in the spirit of recovery is the courage to hope and the willingness to try. This is unlikely to be nurtured by a service that focuses solely on skills. In contrast to this, humanistic care is concerned more with an individual's growth, than cure. It is concerned with creating a social milieu which enables people to move towards what Rogers calls becoming a fully functioning person – a journey which we all share.

A need is a lack of something that, if it remains unsatisfied, expresses itself as suffering. Mosher and Burti put identifying needs at the centre of their model for community mental health services:

> 'In our work we are primarily concerned with needs: we prefer to consider symptoms as communications about unmet needs that may be recognised and met rather than as expressions of hypothetical, underlying pathological processes, whose classification results in little advantage to the patient. We must understand the message in order to recognise the presenting needs; the psychological mechanisms of symptom formation are of less concern to us.' (p. 19)

There have been many attempts to classify human needs. Abraham Maslow, one of the founding fathers of humanistic psychology, developed one of the best known classifications. Our level of well-being can be seen as a barometer of how successful we are in meeting these needs in everyday life. Mental health services users, whose vulnerabilities and social disadvantage keep them on the edge of distress, are people whose wants and needs are often frustrated and remain unmet. What service users say they want is an ordinary life, not a life that is lived within the parameters of a mental health service provision that is annexed from the mainstream of community life. Why should people with mental health problems need a health and fitness centre of their own when there are many perfectly good ones in the locality? Do they have different housing needs from anybody else? They may need support in accessing and using these resources, but that is a different issue.

It is helpful to keep in mind that the needs of a person with a mental health problem are no different from our own. They may be more urgent and pressing, they may be creating more tension and anguish at that moment in time, but in essence they are the same needs that we all have.

Wants can be aspirations that reflect basic human needs. This fits with the stress vulnerability model of mental disorder widely used as a model for understanding and responding therapeutically to the spectrum of distressed and disturbed behaviour that people seek help with.

Human needs
- To be authentic – become the person we are.
- To express our spiritual nature.
- To affiliate and belong.

- To be valued and value ourselves.
- To love and be loved.
- To express our sexuality.
- To feel secure and attached.
- To meet our physiological needs.

(Adapted from Maslow, 1954)

Of course, people do not usually express their needs and wants in quite these terms. The self-assessed needs of mental health service users consistently highlight that what they want is a home; enough money to live on; a meaningful day; support and friends; relief from suffering and access to specialist help (Strathdee *et al.,* 1997). A recent user-led research survey (Mental Health Foundation, 1997) identified the following needs and wants when in distress:

- Someone to talk to.
- Help to manage my feelings.
- Support from someone who will listen to me.
- Help to relax.
- Somewhere to be safe.
- Easier access to psychiatric care when I'm unwell.
- Help with practical problems.
- Help to cope with my voices.
- Information about illness, treatment, services.
- Help with social recovery.
- Spiritual care.
- Acceptance.
- Privacy and peace.
- To be looked after.
- Counselling.
- Medication.
- Complementary therapies.

It might seem that the pursuit of satisfying needs reflects an obsession with self. While narcissism is a necessary phase in development, the meeting of needs in the context of adult relationships becomes more reciprocal and altruistic (Argyle, 1994). In the person-centred approach to helping, the need to feel loved and valued is emphasized as a prerequisite for growth and the unfolding of our potential. As we grow towards being more authentic, more aware and accepting of ourselves, we become more effective in meeting our own needs and become more aware and responsive to the needs of others. There is, for example, often a great deal of anger in the experience of depression. Often people will be unable to own their anger and other feelings that are related to frustrated, unmet needs. Early experience has taught people that the open expression of needs and feelings will meet with disapproval or rejection. They learn that love is conditional on not being needy, not being upset. Disowning needs and feeling becomes a pattern and people no longer know what they need or what they feel, they have become alienated from their authentic selves. For many people, the experience of depression is a grey dawn that settles on the landscape of their lives, robbing it of colour and life. In the profound bleakness of that experience is the despair of ever being prized enough to have their needs and feelings accepted, and anger that this should be so. Sometimes such despair and anger becomes unbearable and the act of suicide the only solace.

Awareness of another's needs is only possible if we can be sensitive and empathic to what the client is saying metaphorically in distressed and disturbed behaviour. If we can we listen to a person's experience as it unfolds, from their frame of reference, so that it is almost as if we are sharing the experience, we can get a sense of what needs underlie their presenting behaviour. For example, a young Anglo-African man was referred to the service with a history of voice hearing. In an effort to be accepted into the host culture he had anglicized his name and limited the expression of his cultural heritage in his life style. His voice hearing began during a period when had been feeling depressed following the death of his mother. The voices were sometimes abusive and taunting, sometimes validating and at times spoke to him in a Nigerian dialect he was not familiar with. He came to interpret these voices as meaning that he was 'special' and 'chosen ' and that he had 'shaman's blood' and began communicating loudly with the spirit world and posting sachets of 'herbal remedies' through the doors of neighbours. This may be seen to be unusual and disruptive expressions of a need to be valued and belong, to be his authentic self in a way that honoured his ethnicity and cultural heritage.

Peplau (1988) has written widely about needs in the context of nursing care. She argues that:

> 'only the patient knows what his needs are and he is not always able to identify them, knowing only that he feels the tension that needs generate. Paying attention to the needs of the patient, so that personalities can develop further, is a way of using nursing as a social force that aids people to identify what they want and to feel free and able to struggle with others to find satisfaction. Progressive identification of needs takes place as nurse and patient communicate with each other in an interpersonal relationship'. (p. 84)

Peplau takes a broadly humanistic view of needs, i.e. that when basic needs are substantially met – our physiological needs, our needs for security, our need for love and belonging and the need to feel valued and to value ourselves – then more of our energy is free to develop our potential as human beings. We then begin to move towards creative, constructive, productive, personal and community living.

Jamie's story *(Theme: a needs approach to care)*
Jamie is a young man who has had numerous referrals to the mental health services. He grew up in a family with a physically abusive father and a depressed mother who had often been hospitalized. The most nurturing relationship in his life was with his grandmother who died when he was eleven. He lives a chaotic lifestyle with no structure or anchor points. He is a sociable person but seems unable to develop relationships beyond a superficial

level. His life is currently punctuated by frequent crises in which he complains of unbearable tension, feels depressed and is wracked by thoughts that he is 'bad through and through'. At times he hears voices telling him to hang himself. The tension is expressed and finds some relief in excessive drinking, drug misuse and self-harm behaviour. During the course of various psychiatric assessments, a number of diagnoses have been made: schizo-affective disorder, personality disorder, drug-induced psychosis complicated by problematic drinking. He now thinks of himself as ill and has become adept at being a psychiatric patient, at getting psycho-active drugs prescribed and at gaining admission where his needs are for a time at least partially met and his tension subsides.

An alternative explanatory hypothesis of Jamie's presenting problems could be that his behaviour is a dramatic and damaging way of expressing and getting some response to his unmet needs. Adopting a needs-led approach to this scenario, Jamie's care co-ordinator will have a central role in helping him identify his needs, articulated in a language that has meaning for him. Through a developing relationship there would be some direct response to these needs and help in accessing other resources. It would be onerous if not impossible for any individual mental health worker sufficiently to meet all of the needs this client has and other sources of support would need to be in place. It is only when he has a secure base provided by relationships with mental health workers, who are able to acknowledge and contain his distress and relate to him in a way that enables him to feel warmly accepted and valued, that he will be able to move on in his development as a person and reclaim an ordinary life. Building a relationship that is different enough to make a difference requires time and commitment. It requires a team or organizational culture in which staff feel supported and have their own feelings of anxiety, despondency, failure, inadequacy, anger that can surface in the care of people like Jamie, acknowledged and contained.

The focus for much of the debate on a needs-led service centres not so much on what we have been discussing so far, the individual needs of service users, but on the availability of resources in a locality to meet the mental health needs of a local population. For example, the need for a 24-hour crisis response service, activity centres, supported housing, family intervention service, counselling services, complementary therapies, intensive care beds, crisis houses, outreach services, and so on. The user movement is becoming increasingly active and influential in the planning and development of services and in setting up alternatives to the statutory and agency provision, in the form of self-help groups, drop-in centres and sanctuaries. There has been some criticism of the community provision taking shape in the UK, which is seen by some service users as the re-invention of the institution in the community in a way that does not address their real needs (Sainsbury Centre, 1997c). The experience of many service users is that their needs are not adequately assessed, particular in relation to the social context of their distress and, as a consequence, the service response is at best only partially helpful. There can be too much emphasis on neuropathology and psychopathology so that people come to believe that the problem is within, rather than the social and economic context in which they live their lives. Assessment of need should be from the user perspective. They should be able to negotiate a care programme that best meets their needs. The danger with a needs-led service that focuses too much on the provision of resources is that people with mental health problems will have to fit into whatever is available. For example, it can become routine practice for someone diagnosed as having schizophrenia to be prescribed depot neuroleptics, to attend a mental health resource centre and receive fortnightly visits by a CPN, who monitors symptoms and side effects and provides support. This may fall far short of the service user's need for better housing, a socially valued way of spending their time, ways of coping with the unusual thoughts and voices that trouble them and a need for an improved relationship with their family. There is a need for professionals, particularly case managers, to be creative and flexible in response to individual users' needs.

One of the most damning criticisms of community care is that it has failed to meet the needs of the most vulnerable service users. Those with long-term disabilities often either slip through cracks in the service or are difficult to engage with. The recognition that the needs of this group were being neglected has led to the setting up of assertive outreach teams. Many people in this group are distrustful of the mental health service as a consequence of previous experience and actively avoid contact. The key to engaging with this group is the ability of the key worker to establish a relationship that is accepting and understanding and seeks to be of practical help.

There has also been criticism of the inadequacy of the provision for users from ethnic minority groups. Services can be very ethnocentric, reflecting Western values of mental health and individual needs. There are concerns about the discriminatory processes in psychiatry which are reflected in the higher diagnostic rates for schizophrenia, more compulsory admissions, high doses of medication and more unmet needs among service users in the ethnic minorities (Fernando, 1995).

People can take responsibility for themselves

A useful adage for humanistic helpers would be *less is more*! The less we can do for someone, the more they are likely to develop a sense of personal power and agency. The aim is to work with people in collaborative and facilitative ways that maximize autonomy and self-help, with the professional helper being the midwife of change, not the originator. 'At the heart of humanistic helping is a belief in the trustworthiness of the person seeking help, as someone capable of evaluating their inner and outer world, understanding himself in its context and make choices as to the next step in life and act on those choices' (Rogers, 1997, p. 382). Brandon (1976), in exploring the art of helping, highlights the damage that professional helpers can do to a person's sense of their own agency if they take over the problems of living that service users face and attempt to deal with human distress in a prescriptive way. Along that therapeutic route we find increasing passivity, dependency and helplessness. It is natural for us as mental health workers to want to do something to relieve distress or to change behaviour that is damaging or limiting, but we can become so impelled by our desire to help that it becomes a kind of craving that makes it difficult for us to tolerate others' distress and accept unwise behaviour. In an interesting exploration of the Buddhist philosophy of helping, Groves (1998) suggests helpers should work at developing the skilful qualities of unconditional lovingkindness and mindfulness. This allows us to be with people in a way that values them, that communicates warm regard, without demanding anything in return. Mindfulness allows us to be more aware of others, to be more aware of ourselves and more aware of the effect of our presence on others. These two qualities when present in the helper can have a liberating effect on people seeking help. If we can stop hindering the recovery process, distress will run its course and the individual will begin to respond to inner prompting to find a way of being in the world that engenders less suffering. This is very similar to the claim made for a person-centred approach to psychological helping, that being with people in a real, empathic, accepting way facilitates growth and resourcefulness, so that among other changes they will:

- Show fewer characteristics normally labelled psychotic or neurotic.
- Become more self-knowledgeable and more accepting of self.
- Become more self-directing and self-confident.
- Become better able to cope with the problems of living more effectively and comfortably (Rogers, 1967).

In his clinical practice, Rogers became convinced that it is always the client who knows what hurts and what direction they need to move in for healing to take place. The helper's task is to aid people to discover their inner resources, not to impose solutions, strategies, explanations and interpretations. When there is a commitment to understanding the subjective world of the clients and the clients feel understood, they begin to move forward in constructive, positive ways (Thorne, 1992). The act of helping then is not only concerned with enabling people to deal in less distressing, problematic ways in the here and now, but should also leave them more resourceful and less vulnerable to the challenges of living they will face in the future.

Empowerment is a word that has been used to wrap professionalized care in an attractive package, but it is a mistake to think that professional helpers can empower anyone. Power has to be taken, it can never be conferred. The best we can do is not block the assertion of autonomy in the ways we relate to people in care. Helpers need to reflect critically on their practice and be watchful of actions that deprive clients of opportunities to develop or assert their autonomy and control. The helping process should be transparent. The French philosopher Foucault argues that power is bound up with knowledge. Experts, particularly experts in the psychiatric professions who claim an understanding of human distress and what to do about it, hold considerable power, power that is sanctioned by society. Psychiatric knowledge is mystifying to those on the outside, which therefore places people using the mental health services in a dependent position. It can be very difficult for an individual to exercise self-determination in an expert-led service that expects compliance. What if the dominant discourses that circulate in society about psychological distress are not absolute truths, but simply hypothetical constructions that offer a keyhole view of the nature of human distress? In recent years the edifice of Freudian psychoanalytic psychology has been exposed as a creative but flawed construction of human experience (Masson, 1988). Similarly the construction of deeply distressed people as ill and in need of treatment rather than care in a healing environment, has been called into question.

Self-determination, choice and self-help are at the heart of individual recovery programmes. Psycho-social distress is not experienced passively. Most people try various strategies to cope with it, with varying degrees of success. Identifying and enhancing those strategies that have worked for individuals and teaching additional strategies can encourage a sense of control over problematic thoughts, feelings and behaviour. In a recent study (Mental Health Foundation, 1997) 80% of people said that they had developed personal ways of coping with aspects of their daily life and experience that were difficult and distressing. People who use the mental health service will have their own ways of motivating themselves, getting support, managing disturbing experiences, coping with crisis and surviving, that should be recognized, respected and encouraged. Some coping strategies can, of course, be damaging and limiting if used excessively, for example withdrawal, self-harming, or the use of alcohol. Individual care planning is concerned with helping people become less reliant on disruptive or harmful strategies through developing and strengthening their repertoire of positive strategies.

Examples of positive coping strategies from a representative group of service users

Complementary therapies, leisure and recreational activities, yoga, physical activity, art and music, relaxation techniques, reading, adult education classes, walks in the countryside, prayer and religious contemplation, using medication, slowing down, expressing my feelings, keeping pets, keeping busy, disputing worrying thoughts, positive affirmation, talking with friends and family, talking with a mental health professionals, joining a self-help group or user group, keeping a journal, listening to talking books, finding out about my mental health problem, contacting the crisis line, helping others, having a socially valued occupation, taking respite breaks, getting enough rest, being listened to, understanding my symptoms motivating myself, taking one day at a time, having a routine, having achievable goals, monitoring my symptoms, avoid overloading myself.

(Source: Mental Health Foundation, 1997)

Many people with long-term mental health problems have benefited from an involvement with self-help and user groups. In most areas of the UK people will now be able to find support groups made up of people with similar difficulties and experiences to their own. Such groups operate to varying degrees outside the statutory mental health service provision, although they may be sponsored and assisted by it. They provide an alternative to professionalized mental health care in which helping is reciprocal and takes place in an egalitarian context. Self-help and user groups are significant sources of support, self-help, empowerment and advocacy. For many people membership provides the seed from which the spirit of recovery grows. Even in consumer organizations such as Survivors Speak Out who have a political agenda and are primarily concerned with influencing change within mainstream psychiatry and in the socio-political context in which users live their lives, individuals experience involvement as empowering and healing (Campbell, 1996).

Recovering from long-term mental health problems requires people to be more in charge of their own lives, to become experts in their own self-care. Of necessity this involves 'non-compliance'. When we consider what mental health service users are unmotivated about, or non-compliant with, it is usually some element in their treatment programme that they do not value for themselves, that has been prescribed by others with little consultative discussion. Until people can dream their own dreams and find their own pathway of recovery, their lives will remain circumscribed by the limited vision of others. Patricia Deegan, a psychologist and herself a service user, put it this way:

> 'To me recovery means that I try to stay in charge of my own life. I don't let my illness run me. Over the years I've worked hard to become an expert in my own self-care. For instance, being in recovery means that I don't just take medication. Just taking medication is a passive stance. Rather I use medication as part of my recovery process. In the same way I don't just go into hospital. Just going into hospital is a passive stance. Rather I use the hospital when I need to. Additionally, over the years, I have learned all kinds of ways to help myself. Sometimes I use medication, therapy, self-help and mutual support groups, friends, my relationship with God, my work, exercise, spending time with nature – all these things help me remain whole and healthy even though I have a disability' (Deegan, 1997, p. 21).

A philosophy of care that places a high value on self-determination and self-responsibility does not mean that a person is in some way at fault for failing to recover and flourish. To do so would fail to recognize the social constraints that operate in the lives of many long-term mental health service users. It would fail to recognize the devastating impact of a serious mental health problem on the self-concept, self-esteem and personal aspirations of the individual. It would fail to recognize the need we all have for sustaining and nurturing relationships in order to live out our potential. Neither does it ignore the reality that at times difficult ethical issues will arise in relation to self-determination, when a decision is made that overrides the wish of service user because they or others are at risk.

Part

2

The working alliance

Introduction

For the past 50 years the literature on psychiatric nursing has emphasized the therapeutic value of the relationship between nurses and people using the mental health services, placing the relationship at the heart of mental health care. It must therefore be a cause of some concern that this is not more widely reflected in current practice. Sullivan (1998) in a review of anecdotal and empirical evidence for the therapeutic relationship in psychiatric nursing concludes that, in many care situations there is limited contact and therapeutic interaction between nurses and the people in their care. Despite this, there remains within the profession a strongly held belief that the essence of mental health nursing is the helping relationship underpinned by a pragmatic philosophy (Barker *et al.*, 1997).

In an earlier study of the work of psychiatric nurses, Cormack (1976) noted the resemblance between what people using the service said nurses contributed to their recovery and what Carl Rogers, the originator of person-centred counselling, identified as the necessary and sufficient conditions for change: a helping relationship in which the helper is able to be with the person seeking help in a way that is empathic, accepting and genuine. That these relational qualities are enabling and valued by service users, continues to be endorsed by research (Sheppard, 1993; Rogers and Pilgrim, 1994). The emphasis here is on a way of being in relationship to people in care, not what mental health professionals might know or do. It is this facilitative contact created by these relational qualities that enables people to set out and then continue on the road to recovery.

The helping relationship can take a number of forms. As Egan (1994) puts it, 'The idea of one perfect kind of helping relationship is a myth. Different clients have different needs and these are met through different kinds of relationship' (p. 48). Clarkson (1995) in her perceptive analysis of therapeutic relationships identifies five characterizing elements: the working alliance; the transference-countertransference relationship; the reparative developmentally needed relationship; the person-to-person relationship; and the transpersonal relationship. While this hypothesis has been forged in the main out of the experience of professional counselling and psychotherapy, it seems to me to have a helpful relevance to all mental health workers. The relationship types are not seen as mutually exclusive but coalesce in the therapeutic process. Part 2 takes the working alliance, the basis for all helping relationships, as its central theme.

Chapter 7 is an exploration of beginnings. Connecting with clients in a way that facilitates a sense of rapport and trust is assisted by maintaining a sensitive awareness of the dynamics that commonly come into play in the beginning phase of the helping relationship.

Chapter 8 outlines a pragmatic, problem management framework within which collaborative helping can take place. It involves working creatively with clients to help them find more effective ways of managing the challenges and opportunities of living. Problems of living are part of the fabric of life. We can never eliminate them but we can learn to manage them in ways that are less problematic, distressing and disabling. The framework offers people a strategy for living more fully and resourcefully. Many people, particularly those with long-term mental health problems, have experienced oppression and disempowerment. Often this has prevented them from being the architects of their own life and has inculcated a sense of helplessness, hopelessness and dependency. Chapter 9 examines the working alliance as an enabling relationship that aims to help clients discover and express their personal power.

In Chapter 10, the working alliance between mental health professionals and their clients is discussed in the context of independent advocacy. Advocacy is seen as having enormous benefit, particularly for clients who have felt discounted, disbelieved, de-valued and disempowered in their dealings with the psychiatric system and the wider social systems that impact on their lives.

In Chapter 11, the role of case manager is explored, a role that many mental health professionals now occupy. Where it works well case management is liked and valued by clients and carers. It is based on a strong working alliance that is concerned not only with facilitating access to resources and services, but also with long-term interactional work with clients, most of whom have complex problems and needs.

Chapter 12 broadens the parameters of the working alliance to include carers and their families. The importance of families in enhancing the well-being of individuals distressed and disabled by enduring mental health problems is recognized and discussed. For families to maintain a social environment in which the recovery process can take place, mental health professionals must address their needs, problems and issues. Despite the best endeavours of mental health professionals, some clients remain difficult to engage and work with. It can take months of persistent effort to forge a tenuous alliance and concordance. This should not come as a surprise. Often the history of service users is of abusive relationships in the personal sphere of their lives and oppressive encounters with health and social services. Chapter 13 considers the issue of non-compliance. Non-compliance should not always be viewed negatively. For some people defending the sovereignty of their lives against the incursions of mental health professionals represents the tender shoots of recovery.

Chapter 14 explores the dynamics of the end phase of the working alliance. Issues triggered by endings can be difficult both for the client and the helper alike and need to be managed with awareness and sensitivity. While the working alliance can be an enabling presence that is a significant factor in the client's recovery process, at some point it must end if we are not to hold people in a co-dependent relationship.

7 Beginnings and the working alliance

Beginnings are important. The foundations are being laid for a working alliance without which it will be difficult to help the client. This phase in the helping process can be brief or it can take some time, but it cannot be rushed. Early impressions fundamentally affect the shaping of the relationship. For instance, mental health nurses who create an initial impression of being controlling or insensitive may find that impression difficult to break down.

Often assumptions and expectations are present before nurse and client come face to face. Clients may have had a bad experience of mental health services in the past. They may have experienced oppressive or unhelpful care. They may resent their referral, which has hence involved an element of coercion. They may be fearful that in becoming involved with the mental health services they will be stigmatized and their personhood submerged by psychiatric patient status. As nurses we may be influenced by a client's reported history or diagnosis and have a prejudiced picture of them before we have even met.

It can be very difficult for some clients to trust professional carers and they may remain guarded and distant and difficult to reach out to. This may be related to traumatizing experiences of parental or statutory care in their early lives. The legacy of such an experience can be a discomfort with closeness and intimacy and a reluctance to trust others with their vulnerability. As Winship (1995) suggests, it can be difficult to accept the concern and care of staff, if caring figures in the patient's past were persecutory. Care may be perceived with suspicion and hostility. Part of the art of psychiatric nursing is to be able to hold psychologically these projected feelings while building a relationship with the client which is safe enough to enable them to re-own and feel less disturbed by persecutory feelings. Clearly, acting out the client's projections through oppressive action will confirm their deepest fears and undermine the foundations of a working alliance.

Where coercion, compulsion or force has been used in relation to admission or treatment, it is important to acknowledge the psychological trauma that such an experience subjects people to. It should be openly discussed with the client and their feelings heard (Campbell and Lindow, 1997). Considerable perseverance can be required to rebuild a basis of trust.

Building trust means going at the client's pace and not pushing so hard that reluctance becomes resistance. In our initial contact with a client, we need to put the emphasis on ourselves as people – the person rather than the role. A client is much more likely to engage with you the individual than you the psychiatric nurse. We need to establish a basis for a collaborative relationship from an early stage by actively seeking the client's views on how they see their needs and what they need help with. Being able to offer some immediate practical help conveys a strong message that you are 'for the client', a potential ally in a world that may seem chaotic, difficult and threatening. It is, however, best to be honest about what you can and cannot offer in terms of direct help and accessing resources. The philosophy of leaving clients with as much power as possible to make choices and decisions, to be in charge of their own lives, needs to come through in the initial interaction. Equally it can be important to give clients permission to rely on the mental health worker at times of difficulty and crisis.

A common concern for clients is, 'Will I be heard? Not just listened to politely but have my disclosures respected and taken seriously?' The experience of severe psychological distress and disturbance can be very alienating and clients will feel a great need to be understood. Many people wish their experience to be understood in personal human terms and not pathologized and labelled. For some clients it is not their psychiatric vulnerability that is their primary concern, but the precariousness of their social circumstances – perhaps the threat of eviction. This therefore needs to be heard and responded to by the nurse if a relationship is going to develop.

With some clients who find it hard to engage with the service, it may be necessary to establish contact through a trusted friend, neighbour or another service user. Sometimes the difficulty in establishing rapport can be due to a social, cultural or gender difference between the client and mental health worker and referring on to a colleague may be necessary to engage a client with the service. This should be seen as a sensitively aware, client-centred strategy and not as an admission of professional failure or inadequacy. There is some evidence that ex-service users employed as project workers within community mental health teams can be effective in gaining the trust of disaffected clients (Sainsbury Centre, 1998a).

You will see from all of this that beginnings frequently require effort and sensitivity. It helps to try to get an early intuitive sense of the client's social receptivity and willingness to engage in the care process. Some clients are receptive to a warm supportive presence. Others respond better to a slightly more 'business-like' approach.

Indications that the relationship has moved beyond the beginning stage will be the sense that the client is more at ease, open and less defensive and when there is a real feeling of connecting. You are no longer meeting as strangers. The client has begun to identify you as someone that can be of help.

Self-enquiry Box

- *Brainstorm a list of words associated with beginnings.*
- *Reflect on the experience of beginnings in your own life.*

8 A framework for the working alliance

The skilled helper model, developed by Gerard Egan (1994) and widely adopted by mental health professionals in the UK, offers a useful framework for the working alliance. It is a model that is at its heart person-centred, collaborative and empowering. Egan takes the view that helping is both a social influence process and a process that values client self-responsibility. Achieving this balance is important if the alliance is not to become coercive, controlling and oppressive.

Democratizing the helping process is encouraged if we can:

- Meet people with humanity and humility so that the alliance is one of equals.
- Acknowledge that as helpers we are both resourceful and fallible, as is the client.
- Recognize that power can be shared, discovered and generated within the helping alliance.
- Make the helping process participative rather than directive.
- Share our knowledge of the helping process so that people can become more resourceful and self-supporting.

Egan's model is essentially a problem management approach to helping (Figure 8.1). He argues that when it comes to personal, relational and social problems, we are not terribly good problem solvers. There is a tendency to put up with difficulties, ignore them, deny them, minimize them, or attempt the same ineffective solutions over and over. Distress, disturbance and disablement build up in the wake of undealt with problems. The helping process is concerned with enabling people to become more resourceful and creative in managing the problems facing them, both in their inner and outer worlds. The helper's task is to engage those seeking help in a process that moves through three stages:

- Helping clients identify and clarify needs and problems.
- Helping clients create a better future.
- Helping clients create strategies to move forward.

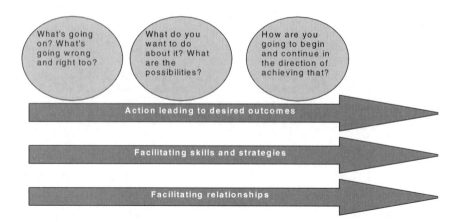

Figure 8.1 The skilled helper model (adapted from Egan, 1994)

Helping clients identify and clarify needs and problems

The first stage of this model is to help the client tell his or her story. Some people will readily seize the opportunity to talk about what is going on and what is going wrong. To unload what might seem daunting, frightening, puzzling or painful experiences to someone who is able to listen supportively can be a great relief. But, given a natural reticence in our culture and an understandable anxiety about the consequences of disclosing personal information, most people need to feel a sense of trust and safety before they are able to share and explore their problems fully. In telling their story the client is often acknowledging and facing difficult and painful issues that may have, until now, been kept at a distance. As the story emerges, the associated emotional distress may surface with it and be discharged. In the exploratory dialogue between the helper and client, the story is filled out and new perspectives can emerge. The issues and problems of living that confront the client can be viewed with more clarity or seen differently. This can mean that a problem might not seem quite so disturbing and distressing – it can be faced and coped with, opportunities can be seen.

As the client's story unfolds we need to try to avoid assumptions and interpretations. Our task as helpers is to come to a shared understanding of the client's reality. We need to know what meaning the term depression has in relation to the client's experience of himself and his life. Words, as Wittgenstein argues, do not describe reality, but create the reality out of experience (Lynch, 1997). Having expert knowledge does not give mental health professionals insight into an individual's reality; the client is the expert on that. Understanding a client's experience comes through finding a common language from which something of the client's world and its meanings can be communicated. Essentially the task of all therapeutic conversation is to find a way of co-creating a different or preferred reality.

Sarita's story *(Theme: identifying and clarifying needs and problems)*

Sarita is a 28-year-old woman who has been diagnosed as having schizophrenia. Despite trying various neuroleptic drugs she struggles to stay free of intrusive and disruptive delusional ideas. The feeling that people are watching and following her surfaces and begins to take hold, as does the belief that CCTV cameras monitor her movements. These distressing thoughts cause her to isolate herself in her flat. She also complains of hearing 'whispering', which she interprets as evidence of the close surveillance she is under.

The dialogue transcribed below took place following an incident in which the police were called to the flats where Sarita lives after neighbours heard her shouting at her persecutors. She has had three previous admissions to an acute psychiatric admission unit, during which she became very depressed and apathetic. The community team is trying to help Sarita manage this crisis episode without resorting to hospitalization.

A CPN has established a working alliance with Sarita in which she feels safe enough to share her experience.

CPN: To believe that you're being watched and followed must be frightening.

Sarita: (crying) I can't go out now. They're always there. Did you see anyone around outside when you arrived? Perhaps I should go back to the hospital?

CPN: I'm sorry you're feeling so upset and unsafe. I didn't see anyone suspicious in the street. Why do you think this is happening to you?

Sarita: They think I'm here illegally, don't they and they're trying to get rid of me. I've seen the cameras in the town picking me out of the crowd. Just because I've had this mental trouble they want to get rid of me.

CPN: Are you saying that because you've had some psychiatric problems over the past few years you think the police and the immigration people have been told to get rid of you?

Sarita (nods): That's why they were here today.

CPN: Can you think of any other explanation for why the police came? How would it seem if I said that they were called because someone here heard you shouting and they were concerned about you and didn't know what else to do?

Sarita: They couldn't give a fuck about me. I've heard them say they ought to put her in hospital or pack her off home.

CPN: That must feel pretty hurtful.

CPN: This worry about being watched and followed – is that something that's on your mind a lot, or just from time to time?

Sarita: They could come and get me any time. I can't sleep because they might come at night when it's quiet.

CPN: Do you think you need to be in hospital?

> Sarita: Part of me does. I'd feel safer there. They can't touch me there you see, there are too many witnesses. But I'm afraid I will lose myself if I go in again. I don't want to end up one of those empty-eyed women.
>
> CPN: You feel like you might, in a way, lose any chance of a normal life if you go in again? You seem a bit calmer since we've been talking and I'm wondering how it would be for you if I called more frequently over the next few days and Janice (housing project worker) spent more time with you? Would that help you feel safer?
>
> As Sarita's story unfolds it seemed that these unusual thoughts were linked in some way to her experience of discrimination both as an Asian woman and as a user of the mental health service. Her family are Ugandan Asians who were forced to leave Uganda during Idi Amin's oppressive regime. They were subjected to a great deal of intimidation prior to their exclusion and arrived in Britain as political refugees with very little. Although they had legal citizenship and have now created a new life for themselves, a legacy of insecurity and distrust has persisted in the family culture. Sarita's mother appeared to suffer from a disabling post-traumatic stress disorder for several years after the family's arrival in the UK. As a young woman Sarita's Westernized values, a failed marriage to a white Englishman and in recent years her mental health problems, have progressively alienated her from her family. This alienated, depressed state of mind seemed to allow persecutory thoughts to surface, take hold and take on a more extreme form. Enabling Sarita to tell her story within the context of a safe and supportive relationship relieved some of the emotional tension and distress that had built up around her disturbing thoughts and gave meaning to them. It also opened up possibilities for helping her manage this vulnerability more effectively, without the need for increasing medication or admitting her to hospital.

Often the problems of living that people seek help with from the mental health services are quite complex. As a story unfolds there may be a history of abuse in childhood, problem drinking, low self-esteem, volatile moods, debts, housing difficulties, suicide attempts. Egan argues that to try to work on all fronts can be overwhelming for the client and the helper. Priorities need to be identified. What is the client motivated to do something about? What would make a significant difference to their sense of well-being? Unless there is a shared perception about what the problems and needs are that the client could use help with, then the helping process will stall at the outset. This is not to say that as helpers we should collude with clients to avoid the difficult and challenging issues they face. We should make reasonable demands and encourage people to make reasonable demands on themselves. Egan identifies a number of principles for getting leverage in helping people manage their problems in living:

- If there is a crisis, first help the client manage the crisis.

- Begin with the problem that causes most distress.
- Begin with the issue that the client sees as important, which may be different from the helper's assessment.
- Begin with a manageable part of the problem. Problem management is often incremental, involving small steps rather than giant strides.
- Begin with a problem that will lead to an overall improvement in well-being.

Finding a different way of being that is less problematic and overcoming social disadvantage and adversity, are not easy tasks. Sometimes problems can seem to defy efforts to resolve them and create a stagnant pool of powerless and helplessness. At times it can be better to surrender to a problem, to stop working so hard to resolve it. Surrendering does not mean passively resigning oneself to a life limited by a problem or its negative effects, it means letting go of the tension that builds up around frustrated attempts at resolution. Sometimes this release of pressure opens up new possibilities. A new-found acceptance of personal vulnerabilities emerges, leading to creative ways of managing and transcending them. On the other hand, many people who seek the help of mental health services readily retreat into helplessness when faced with the difficulties of living. For those individuals, the need is one of asserting some control over problem situations rather than surrender. Their learnt helplessness needs to be replaced by the discovery of their resourcefulness. Through engaging people in a problem management process, a sense of being more in control of one's life begins to emerge, which can be both freeing and empowering.

Creating a better future

The second stage of Egan's problem management process is concerned with helping the client construct a better future. In other words, it is concerned with exploring the possibilities and setting goals, which then become a direction for wise action. The stories that people tell are often problem-saturated. This can so easily be reinforced by mental health professionals if the focus of their interest is solely on dysfunctional aspects of the client's life and does not also bring out their resources and talents. The meaning the client is likely to draw from that problem-saturated perspective, is that they are ill, helpless, hopeless, inadequate or weak and have no future – a bleak picture indeed and one that can trap people in a 'career' as a mental patient or as a victim.

This can be an exciting and satisfying phase in the helping process. People begin to transcend their disabilities and regain a measure of hopefulness and resourcefulness and step out on the road of recovery. Step by step they begin to re-enter life and manage their lives more effectively. In so doing their personal narratives become less problem-saturated and they begin to see themselves in more positive ways. Of course this is not an easy process – a client may well find it easier to adopt the passive role of the ill patient or the victim. Recovering or discovering a sense of personal agency, the sense of being in charge of their own lives, can perhaps be the most difficult part of all of the helping process for people with long-term mental health problems, since they may have an understandable tendency to retreat from the significant and distressing problems of living into passivity, helplessness and hopelessness. Unfortunately, disempowering relationships with mental health professionals can compound this protective but ultimately limiting strategy.

This part of the helping process involves asking future orientated questions, which are intended to identify the possibilities for change. We are asking people to imagine a different life for themselves. Not a fairy tale, happy ever after sort of life, but one in which there is more psychological comfort and social ease than there is now. In doing this we need to be careful that it is the client's wishes that are identified and not our own aspirations for the client based on our own values. It is easy unintentionally to influence clients in the direction of certain goals. For some clients, greater social participation and integration may not be a desired outcome. For others, a higher level of independence may not be a valued goal, although we might value both these behavioural characteristics for ourselves.

The following are useful future-orientated questions that you may find helpful to build into your dialogue with clients. The intention is to stimulate the client's imagination in the search for possibilities, some of which then become the goals for recovery. You will notice that that they are framed in a positive, expectant way – 'When you're coping better', not 'If you were coping better'.

'When you're coping a bit better, what will be happening in your life that's not happening now?'

'How will you know that some improvement is beginning to take place?'

'What will be the first thing you'll notice when you begin to get out from under this depression?'

'When you're beginning to get yourself "sorted out" what changes would others notice?'

'When you're beginning to feel a bit better, what will this enable you to do that you don't do now?'

'What do you want to happen (that would make a difference)?'

'What do you need (that would make a difference)?'

'If a miracle happened and you woke up one morning and this problem had disappeared, what would you notice that was different about you, what would other people notice?'

'Are any parts of this miracle happening already?'

'Tell me about the times when it's not so bad. What's your life like?'

'On a scale of 1–10, with 1 being the worst it's ever been, where would you say you were today? How would you need to be feeling, what would you need to be doing, to have moved up the scale a couple of points?'

'If you were able to get a pill for any characteristic, e.g. for confidence, which pills would you ask for? How would that make a difference to your life?'

Egan has suggested that, for many clients, it is helpful to engage in future-orientated, solution focused talk early in the helping process. Pursuing a lengthy search of a person's history in the hope that insight and re-evaluation will lead to liberation from a problematic past and automatically enable people to create a better future for themselves, is not particularly helpful. Talking endlessly with a client about the story of their disruptive highs and disabling lows gets nowhere, but if we can engage them in a dialogue about possibilities, e.g. 'What will be happening when you are managing this problem better?' some hopefulness, direction and motivation can return. Possible replies might then be:

'I would be able to hold down a job.'

'I wouldn't have to take so much medication.'

'I would be steadier in my mood.'

'I would have a better relationship with my family.'

'I would feel better about myself, not so useless.'

'My life wouldn't feel so empty.'

If it seems helpful, more exploratory work can be done on the story in the light of these possibilities – 'Could you say some more about how family relationships have been affected?' From these broad statements that the client makes about his preferred future, more specific goals can be teased out: 'What would you have in your life that you don't have now if it didn't feel so empty?' 'I would like you to notice what's happening in your life on those occasions when you do feel a bit better about yourself?' Of course, clients often do not find it easy to respond to future-orientated questions. They may be so sunk in their problems, feel so pessimistic and disempowered that the future is difficult to imagine. It can require considerable encouragement and an attitude of realistic optimism from the nurse to enable some clients to become active in this part of the process. Sometimes it can help for clients to notice things that happen that make life a little better and that they would like to keep on happening.

Possibilities translate into goals or desired outcomes that, when realized, would represent some positive change in the client's well-being. They need to be realistic and reachable. Goals may need to be broken down into smaller steps, e.g. obtaining a place on a supported employment programme, before attempting to re-enter the job market. The client must feel a sense of commitment to their goals. It is just no good if the goals 'belong' to someone else.

For some people, leaving the sanctuary of a problem-filled life can be difficult. It might seem inappropriate to use the term sanctuary in connection with enduring mental health problems that can impose such limits on a person's life. Yet it is precisely because of those imposed limitations that they are sometimes difficult to give up. To move towards becoming a fully functioning person, more engaged in living, means facing the struggles of everyday life with all its pleasures, pains and responsibilities.

It can also be equally difficult for some mental health professionals to allow people to choose that struggle. Looking openly with clients at the gains and the losses that are likely to occur as a consequence of moving towards a goal can be helpful. This process can be similar to a balance sheet – if the losses outweigh the gains, a person is unlikely to be motivated to move in the direction of a desired outcome. However, goals can be strongly motivating – many survivors have made heroic efforts to reclaim lives that have been severely damaged by long-term mental health problems and what Breggin (1993) calls toxic psychiatry. Once some goals are established, we can then think about the bridges that need to be built to help the client move from their present position to where they would like to be.

Sarita's story continued *(Theme: creating a better future)*
The following conversation took place between Sarita and her CPN after she had managed to get a good night's sleep.

CPN: What do you feel you need at the moment that would make things a bit better for you?

Sarita: I just want it to stop. I want them to leave me alone.

CPN: Not to be worried by thoughts that the police are going to arrive and arrest you and send you away somewhere? You need to feel safe?

Sarita : Yes. But they're not ordinary police. You can't tell who they are. I think they are like a secret force that no one knows about. I can't get any peace if they're whispering at me. I know Dr Parkes said it was because I was ill, but I can hear them.

CPN: I'm sure they seem very real to you. One thing I notice though is that I can faintly hear people talking in the flat next door and downstairs and I can hear their televisions. I wondered if some of the time that's what you hear?

Sarita: It could be I suppose, but I hear them when I'm not here sometimes.

CPN: So what would help you feel a good deal better would be if those thoughts about being watched and arrested were not bothering you so much and if the whispering stopped?

CPN: When you have got these worries sorted out what will life be like for you?

Sarita: I don't know. I suppose I will go back to The Beeches (a resource centre). It's all right there, but I would like to have a job. I haven't worked since I got ill.

CPN: What will be good about having a job?

Sarita: I would have some money and be able to get some decent clothes. It would mean having a normal life again. I would quite like to finish my business studies course as well. That would please my father.

CPN: Would it please you?

Sarita : Yes it would, but I would probably have to start again and I haven't done any studying for years. I don't know if my mind's strong enough really.

CPN: Are you also thinking it would be a way of reconnecting with your family?

Sarita: I would like to have more contact with them, but when I spoke to my mother a couple of weeks ago she said that I shouldn't come because my father has been unwell. He has diabetes, you see, and heart trouble. The doctor has said he shouldn't have any stress.

CPN: How did you feel after that conversation with your mother?

Sarita: I felt upset at the time. A bit angry really. It was as if they didn't care about me any more. I feel like I've been banished.

CPN: A bit like those thoughts you have about being arrested and thrown out of the country?

CPN: It sounds as if one of the things that would make a difference to your life would be if you were able to be closer to your family again?

This conversation with its future orientation led to some realistic outcomes being identified that would, when they were in place, make a significant difference to Sarita's sense of well-being and the problems she experiences in living. These included:

1. Be able to deal with thoughts about being watched and followed so that they are no longer so intrusive or upsetting.
2. Be able to deal with thoughts of being arrested and deported so they are no longer so troubling.
3. Stop the experience of hearing people whispering.
4. Improve relationships with other tenants.
5. Explore the possibilities of getting on to a supported work project.
6. Explore the possibility of access courses to higher education.
7. Re-establish regular telephone and letter contact with my family.

These outcomes can be seen as short-term goals (1–4) and intermediate goals (5–7) which can lead to the realization of longer-term goals: returning to full-time work; returning to higher education studies; re-uniting with her family. Helping Sarita begin to imagine a better future for herself had an immediate effect on her mood and outlook, with not just her vulnerabilities being addressed in the dialogue but also her abilities and the possibilities in her life.

Creating strategies to move forward

Many clients are already employing helpful strategies to deal with the problems they face in living. Barrowclough and Tarrier (1997), commenting on the findings of studies of coping behaviour in people diagnosed as having schizophrenia, conclude that the majority of people develop coping strategies with varying degrees of success. In a similar study of people who experience manic depression, 62% of respondents recognized the value of self-management strategies and were able to use these to some extent (Hill *et al.*, 1996). It is therefore important to recognize that people are not passive victims of their mental health problems but fight back against them in many ways. Acknowledging how people have been coping reinforces resourcefulness and encourages them to continue their efforts to manage their problems. Research into coping strategies enhancement carried out by Tarrier *et al.* (1993) indicates the value of strengthening current coping behaviour and teaching clients new and different strategies in overcoming persistent disabilities.

Interventions drawn from solution-focused therapy can be effective in helping clients find strategies to move forward in their recovery (Mason *et al.*, 1994; Wilgosh *et al.*, 1994). Clients are helped to identify current strategies by asking solution-focused questions:

'Are there times when you don't let the voices "take over your mind?" How do you do that?'

'So there are some days when despite feeling bad you manage to get up and get on with the day. What happens that helps you manage that?'

'So on a scale of 0–10, with 0 being the worst you've ever been, you feel you're around 3. What's helped you get from 1 to 3? What would you need to do to move up to 5?'

Genuinely complimenting clients on their efforts to overcome their problems emphasizes strengths not weaknesses, competencies not deficits, solutions not problems. The client is acknowledged as the 'expert' on their own problems in living, with the nurse then collaborating with them to find ways of using their own strategies more effectively. Some clients may find it hard to identify helpful ways of getting to where they want to be, so that helpers may need to bring some energy to the process of searching out 'best fit' strategies just as they helped to identify goals. They may often need to make suggestions or to provide information, but this needs to be done in a collaborative way that allows the client to decide if it is right for them. Exploring possible ways forward can involve asking questions such as:

'Do you have any thoughts about what helps you most when you feel particularly vulnerable like this?'

'What are some of the ways you might deal with this?'

'Have you spoken with anyone else that has this problem? How did they deal with it?'

'When you feel bothered by this idea that someone is putting thoughts in your mind, is there anything you can do that helps?'

'You say some days you cope better than others. What helps you to do that?'

'What skills do you think you need to build up to be able to get your own place to live?'

'These times when despite feeling the pressure building up inside your head you don't cut yourself – what do you do or what happens that stops you?'

'Let's think about what you might do that would help you stay OK if you reduced your medication?'

'What help would you like from me (us)? How would that support you?'

This last question is important and one that is seldom asked. We often assume that we know what clients need from us as nurses, but this may not be how they perceive or prioritize their own needs, or what they actually want from their contact from with us. Asking the question encourages self-advocacy.

Like goals, strategies should be realistic, specific and owned by the client. Some people may play it safe and need encouragement to be more adventurous in choosing and using strategies. For strategies to be acted on, it may be necessary to help the client develop an action plan, identifying how, where and when something will be carried out. There is also a danger that, at times, an element of collusion may creep into the relationship between the nurse and client, maintaining a high level of dependence. Other clients may be unrealistic or act blindly, using strategies that are unwise or beyond their present level of competence. For example, a socially isolated young man being supported by the community mental health team, chose to tell people that he met in his local pub and at the filling station where he is a forecourt attendant about his psychiatric history. This led to more rejection, discrimination and a greater sense of isolation. Because of his strong need to feel included, he was inappropriately self-disclosing, so he needed to be more discreet and selective about whom he told.

Sometimes in reviewing their goals with their key worker a client may decide they are unachievable at the present time and there needs to be an intermediate step. A client who was very keen to move on from 24-hour staffed accommodation to a flat of his own in a supported housing project realized that to achieve this goal, he needed to build up his 'self-soothing' skills. He needed to deal with episodes of anxiety that increased his voice hearing so that he could avoid recurrent crises in an environment where he did not have immediate access to staff support.

Sarita's story continued *(Theme: creating strategies to move forward)*

The community team continued to work intensively with Sarita over the following week during which time she began to feel safer and less preoccupied with her unusual beliefs. The therapeutic conversation between Sarita and her CPN is pragmatic and solution focused, concerned with establishing some strategies that will help her manage her disturbing thoughts more effectively. The intensity of face-to-face dialogue is an uncomfortable experience for Sarita, so much of the interaction transcribed below took place during some shared activity.

CPN: When you've had these upsetting thoughts in the past, what's helped, apart from medication?

Sarita: Well I usually have to go into hospital when I really get ill.

CPN: What is it about being in hospital that helps?

Sarita: Having other people around I suppose. I feel safer. I know they won't try anything with so many witnesses. And I can just stay in the ward. I don't have to go out.

CPN: So being with others and sort of hiding yourself away helps you feel safer and less upset. Does talking about these fears you have help?

Sarita: I was worried last time that if I talked about it too much they might give me more drugs. So I kept a lot of it to myself. I remember one nurse used to ask whether it was still on my mind. She used to say that if they were true, the police would have had no trouble in detaining me long before now. So I began to think maybe I had been mistaken and was worrying unnecessarily. She also used to let me help her write the reports in my notes. I'd got this idea in my head at that time that the reports contained coded messages about me that the immigration people would use to deport me. I felt a lot more trusting towards her after that.

Do you think she was right that they would have picked me up by now if they were going to?

CPN: I do, and maybe that's something you can remind yourself about when these ideas begin to get a grip on you.

One of the things that occurs to me is that when you get these thoughts about being watched and followed, you get worried and upset and the more upset you get, the more you have those thoughts. So I'm wondering if there's anything you could do that would help you stay calm. Telling yourself that it can't be true because if the police wanted to pick you up they could do so easily and they haven't, is one useful thing you can do. But I'm wondering if it might also help to tell someone when you notice yourself beginning to think more about being watched or followed. Tell someone at an earlier stage. Not wait until it feels totally real and begins to disrupt your life.

You could phone me and maybe tell Janice (housing project worker). It seems to me that you need someone to reassure you that you're safe at these times. How does that seem to you?

Sarita: I suppose part of me worries that people will think I'm mad. I mean I know it's a sort of illness but I just want a normal life back

CPN: I don't think you're mad but I do think you're very vulnerable to these disturbing thoughts at the moment and if we can help you find some ways of managing them better, you will be able to get your life back on track again. I seem to remember you telling me once that you had got quite good at yoga at one time. I'm thinking that maybe the breathing exercises you learnt might be something else that you could make use of in helping yourself stay calm.

This and other conversations identified a number of cognitive and behavioural strategies that Sarita was encouraged to use to help manage her unusual thoughts and voices and stay in recovery:

- Remind myself that if the police wanted to pick me up they could have done so before.
- Remind myself that surveillance cameras, rather than being a threat, increase my safety.
- Remind myself that voices whispering in the background may be other residents' televisions.
- Concentrate on my breathing exercises if I feel myself getting tense.
- Play some music that is loud enough to drown out the voices without disturbing neighbours.
- Telephone my key worker or project worker at any time if I'm feeling unsafe.

For many clients, following this problem management process through a number of times not only helps them develop strategies for managing or resolving current problems, but also enables them to be more effective when faced with problems in the future. This can be a valuable asset in staying on the road to recovery. However, there will be some clients who will continue to need support in working through the process. Even though they have acquired better problem solving skills, they become easily stressed and continue to need help and encouragement in deciding what to do and when to act on their decision. This need not of course involve a nurse. The support might more helpfully come from an independent advocate, a friend, or a support worker.

The working alliance as an enabling relationship

9

Many clients who seek the help of the mental health services are strongly motivated to seek change in themselves and their lives. Their psycho-social distress requires some relief or resolution. But for many others any movement towards a less problematic life is elusive and they remain immobilized by inertia. This is not meant to strike an overly pessimistic note in relation to the likely outcome of the therapeutic alliance, but much more an encouragement to mental health workers to strike an attitude of realistic optimism in their work.

Passivity colours human behaviour in a number of ways. Most commonly we recognize it as doing nothing when faced with the problems of living. Secondly, we see passivity in compliance – the uncritical acceptance of the understandings and goals suggested by others. Pathologizing psycho-social distress is an 'invitation to infirmity' (Gergen, 1990). If the vulnerabilities and disabilities the client faces are seen as a manifestation of some complex neurophysiological dysfunction, then they resign themselves to being the passive recipients of treatment, often with little hope of recovery. Thirdly, passivity is reflected in purposeless, aimless action. Finally, it can be seen in withdrawal and 'shut down' behaviour.

Deegan (1995) suggests that any passivity, inertia or apathy adopted by people with serious mental health problems is often a defence against the world in which caring about themselves and their lives or being hopeful is too risky – it is safer not to care. Small wonder then that there is a reluctance to emerge from a cocoon of apathy. It is important that nurses involved with the client are able to 'hold' care and hope for that person, until they are able to embrace it for themselves. It is all too easy to give up on people when any change seems a long time coming.

The concept of learnt helplessness, based on the work of Seligman (1975), has established itself in the literature. It hypothesizes passive behaviour as a learnt response to the experience of being faced with life situations over which a person has no influence or control. In such situations, passivity becomes the learnt response and a fixed pattern of behaviour. Once established, even in circumstances to which a person could respond in a way that would make a difference, they do nothing. They are a prisoner of helpless passivity. Deegan (1992) argues that learned helplessness occurs as the consequence of the cycle of disempowerment and despair experienced by many users of the mental health services (Figure 9.1). It expresses itself in apathy,

Attitudinal Barrier
*People with psychiatric
vulnerabilities are
incapable of reasoned
thought and wise action*

The Prophecy is Fulfilled
*Increasing helplessness
dependency and despair*

The System Takes Control
*Professionals take
responsibility*

Learnt Helplessness

Figure 9.1 Cycle of disempowerment and despair

hopelessness, compliance, withdrawal, anxiety, depression and anger, characteristics often interpreted as negative symptoms of schizophrenia and treated with cocktails of powerful neuroleptic drugs. The central issue here is the belief that a psychiatric vulnerability necessarily means that the capability of a person for reasoned thought and wise action is diminished and therefore mental health workers must take that responsibility for them. Many psychiatric survivors argue that this can be more damaging than their psychiatric vulnerability. Disempowering attitudes are not simply found within inpatient services – a legacy of institutional psychiatry – but are also found within community services and in wider society. People with long-term mental health problems are not only marginalized and stigmatized by the nature of their problem, but are also excluded by unemployment and poverty. As mental health professionals, we must try to comprehend the impact on a person of such uncaring social exclusion, which leaves them with one identifiable social role: that of mental patient.

The antidote to learned helplessness requires an attitudinal shift at an individual and organizational level, so that people with disabilities can enter into true partnerships with mental health nurses. They can increasingly become experts in their own care and de-medicalize their lives, instead of becoming experts at occupying a dependent sick role.

We are often very good at sabotaging ourselves with what Egan refers to as disabling self-talk. Often our inner critic will render us speechless and passive in situations that call for a response. This self-imposed impotence gradually undermines our self-confidence and social effectiveness and leads to us avoiding life. Disabling self-talk can be a particular problem for people with enduring or recurrent mental health problems. The recent work of Tarrier on cognitive approaches has become very influential in the field of mental health care, the essence of which is that automatic thoughts and thinking errors have a profound effect on the way we feel and act. If I think I will appear foolish to others, I'm likely to feel anxious about being in the company of others and will avoid socializing. Interventions made by the mental health professional can helpfully focus on assisting clients to identify and dispute these unreasonable thoughts, replacing them with more adaptive ways of thinking. What is being argued is that engaging people in an alliance that is empowering often involves overcoming disabling self-talk.

Power can be seen as a social construction as well as coming from within. Authority and power are invested in social roles to varying degrees. The power that an individual is able to exert in a given situation may depend on factors such as age, gender, social class, education, ethnicity, knowledge and occupational status. The implication of the social construction of power is that its shadow side, oppression, is not a matter of individual attitudes but that it is embedded in social systems. The therapeutic system enshrines this power difference which can be experienced as oppressive and disempowering by clients. McCleod (1998) argues that there are a number of mechanisms at work in therapeutic encounters that are far from empowering in their effect.

The language of psychiatric practice wraps human experience in a blanket of mystifying and excluding terminology, creating the role of expert – one who knows – and the role of client who is the passive recipient of that expertise. Foucault, whose ideas have been influential on the thinking of psychiatric practitioners and user groups, was very interested in the relationship between knowledge and power and, in particular, the knowledge base of the human sciences and the power that acts on human beings. He argued that if there is no such thing as absolute truth, what then is knowledge? It could be the ideas of a powerful minority who impose their views on the majority. The propagation of these views becomes the 'dominant discourse' in society and they are accepted as truths. Those who originate those 'truths' then have a claim to be experts on the behaviour of the rest of us. If certain human experiences are labelled depression and are understood as a neurotransmission deficiency, we are likely to wait passively for the medication to work. If the same human experience is seen as a dispirited state, a consequence of significant loss or of social deprivation, oppression or entrapment, then reviving the spirit and assisting that person to reconnect with their personal power becomes the focus for helping. It also demystifies and deprofessionalizes helping and healing, locating it in the family, the community and society.

A continuing debate has taken place within the mental health professions over the last decade on the issue of empowerment (Gibson, 1991; McDougall, 1997; Campbell and Lindow, 1997). Successive reports have emphasized the need for a partnership in care between professional helpers and clients – *Working in Partnership* (1994), *Pulling Together* (1997). Yet despite this, a service that truly empowers its users still seems an aspiration rather than a reality. The legacy of institutional attitudes persists among many mental health professionals and the medical model still dominates the understanding and management of psychiatric illness. This baggage is less likely to be carried by mental health workers involved in projects run by agencies such as MIND, and it seems likely that the rolling trend towards multi-agency working will enable the philosophy of empowerment to flourish. In addition, the strengthening voice of the user movement and the development of an advocacy network are challenging mental health professionals to rethink their role and philosophy of care.

The term empowerment suggests that it is something that can be given. This is misleading. Empowerment is not a strategy or an intervention but a fundamental way of thinking (McDougall, 1997). It is perhaps more accurate to say that we can facilitate empowerment by not putting barriers in its way through our attitude and our approach to service users and by respecting and nurturing self-esteem, confidence and assertiveness. But, ultimately, mental health workers cannot empower clients, only clients can empower themselves. This means service users accepting more responsibility for themselves in facing the problems and opportunities of living, which can be extremely challenging to many clients whose self-esteem and confidence are low and who, because they have never achieved a strong sense of their own autonomy and initiative, seek out 'the rescuer' in the form of professional helpers when life becomes challenging. This sense of powerlessness is exacerbated by the medicalization of vulnerability and disability. Having a psychiatric diagnosis, particularly of schizophrenia, exposes people to what the user movement has referred to as 'mentalisms' – assumptions that are commonly made about people who are labelled mentally ill (see self-enquiry box). Some appear under a cloak of benevolence, but all are ultimately dehumanizing and disempowering.

Self-enquiry Box

Common mentalisms

The common assumptions outlined below continue to influence the work of mental health professionals. Consider your own response to these statements:
People who have been diagnosed with mental illness:

- *Are likely to be dangerous to themselves and others.*
- *Are likely to need long-term professionalized care if they are to lead ordinary lives.*
- *Are different from me.*
- *Are disabled people, rather than people with disabilities.*
- *Normally do not know what help they need or what is in their best interest.*
- *Are mostly incapable of reasoned thought about their problems. What they say can largely be ignored.*
- *Are mostly not capable of exercising good judgement in making choices and taking decisions.*
- *Are vulnerable people who should be protected from risk and failure.*
- *Often need asylum from mainstream society.*

Why is it that after all this debate many mental health professionals find it difficult to embrace the philosophy of empowerment? The reasons are complex. It is argued (Horsfall, 1997) that many nurses themselves do not feel empowered or supported in their role as care coordinators and primary nurses and may feel unable to express assertively their professional autonomy, particularly if that involves challenging the system. If judicious risk taking is not supported by management, and at times the philosophy of empowerment will entail some risk, nurses may feel unable to allow clients the dignity of risk. At a deeper level, underlying the misuse of power, may be the projection of our own vulnerability and dependency on to clients who then appear more in need of prescriptive care than they actually are. In the background to all this is the fear of litigation if things go wrong, leading to a cautiousness that may limit user choice.

We, as professional mental health workers, may at times feel powerless in our role for a complexity of reasons that may be both related to our personal history and socially constructed.

Caitlin's story *(Theme: nurses' experience of powerlessness)*

Introduction

Caitlin is a recently qualified mental health nurse working in an acute inpatient unit.

I suppose I've never felt a very powerful person, although sometimes clients will say they see me as self-assured, so I must mask it quite well. There are some situations in which I can literally feel my power drain away. Sometimes people's problems and needs seem so enormous and intractable that my contact with them leaves me feeling helpless and inadequate. It seems as if I have little to offer that will make any tangible difference. The supervision I have doesn't help me with that because my supervisor is such a capable and experienced nurse, who always seems to have the 'answers', that it leaves me feeling even more inadequate by comparison.

Meetings and case conferences are also situations in which I lose my voice and often don't say what I want to say. I often end up feeling quite compromised and dissatisfied after meetings. I think it's partly anxiety about challenging authority figures, but also about not really valuing my own point of view highly enough. I suppose I tend to regard most other people as being more able and knowledgeable than I am. I trace this back to my early life and growing up in a male-dominated family in which my mother seemed to defer to my father on most things. She didn't really have an opinion of her own on anything. Although my two brothers were younger than I was, I realized at quite an early age that their achievements were always going to be valued more than mine were. I didn't bother with sixth form and gave up the idea of going to university. I got married instead and started to turn into my mother. In some ways I can identify with the powerlessness many of my clients feel, particularly the women.

Although I still do struggle to hold on to my power in some situations, becoming a psychiatric nurse has been a real emancipation for me. I am feeling more liberated and able to be myself. I do speak my mind a lot more than I used to. I think that power has got to come from within. When I first began to find my voice it sounded quite angry and I really didn't like the way I sounded. I was playing old scripts and expecting to be disregarded or put down and was already resenting it. But because people heard and respected what I had to say, I began to respect myself more. It's been an important lesson that I've tried to take into my work with clients.

Self-enquiry Box

You might like to consider some of the following questions in relation to your own powerlessness.

- *How do I disempower myself?*
- *What is it about this person/this situation/people like this that causes me to lose my power?*
- *How do I empower myself?*
- *How do the social systems, e.g. clinical team, professional discipline, of which I'm part, influence my sense of personal power?*
- *How do the wider social systems, e.g. class, ethnicity, education, affect my sense of personal power?*
- *To what extent does the gender bias in the way power is held, influence my sense of personal power?*
- *Are there times when it is helpful to share my feelings of powerlessness with a client?*
- *Are there times when the feeling of disempowerment I experience belongs to the client?*
- *Do I hold clients in a powerless position to increase my own sense of power?*
- *Do I ever abuse power to cover a sense of powerlessness?*
- *Can I allow myself to feel powerless sometimes?*
- *What can I learn from my experience of powerlessness that can help me understand my client's experience?*

Empowerment may be defined as a process whereby people assert more control over the factors that affect their lives. Connelly *et al.* (1993) suggest that empowerment takes place at a number of levels. In the case of people with enduring mental health problems using the service, this may mean anything from participating in their own care planning by identifying and stating the things they need help with, seeking information and choosing strategies and services that best meet their needs. It also means recognizing and maximizing their talents and personal resources. At the next level, people may feel empowered enough to be of help to others, offering practical help – shopping or form filling, or help in the form of listening or befriending. People often feel a sense of acceptance from peers that is missing from professional relationships. As a sense of personal power grows, people are able to negotiate with others from a position of mutual respect. This may express itself in questioning medication, expressing a view of their needs that differs from that of the professional helpers and being able to agree an acceptable outcome. Some service users and ex-users who feel empowered to this level become independent advocates, or are active in user groups and patient councils. To re-establish a life that has purpose and some measure of satisfaction, in which people are resourceful enough to cope with the challenges and opportunities of living, some progress through these levels of empowerment needs to be achieved.

Empowerment is not of course a one-way process. It can be seen as a continuum, with people sometimes, perhaps during periods of crisis, relinquishing a degree of their autonomy. Empowerment may not always be an entirely positive experience for the client: some clients find the stress of choice and responsibility difficult to bear and need the support of more authoritative relationships. A number of people with high level needs will require 24-hour care in an environment that offers a high level of support and advocacy. Heron (1990), in his Six Category Intervention Analysis model, emphasizes the need for flexibility and judgement in the helping relationship between the poles of authoritative interventions at one end and facilitative interventions at the other (see self-enquiry box). He argues that in our desire to move away from a hierarchical authoritative approach towards facilitative helping, we have thrown out the positive elements with the damaging ones. A client so distressed by unusual and frightening thoughts that he is intent on jumping off a road bridge needs (for a time) care that is both prescriptive and supportive. There is within us all a need for dependency as well as a need for autonomy, which will fluctuate through the life cycle. As Sheehy (1997) puts it, we have a need to separate and achieve a sense of mastery in our world, which she calls *our seeker self* and also a need to merge with others and seek the security and support, our *merger self*. We will return to this theme when we consider developmentally needed relationships. Egan takes up this theme in exploring social influence in the helping process. He suggests that helping exists along a continuum with, for example, a helper insisting on a daily visit to a depressed, at-risk, client's home at one end and respecting client's desire to normalize their life by having only minimal contact with their key worker, at the other. Again judicious flexibility is a key skill in mental health work.

Paul's story *(Theme: disempowerment)*
Being ill, having schizophrenia has made me nervous of people. I'm afraid they will know I have mental trouble even if I don't say anything about being ill, so I don't go out much, just to the clubhouse. When I was in hospital, the nurses used to write things down about you in the report and sometimes they hadn't even spoken to you that day. I remember once feeling that everyone's eyes were following me, it was the worst thing I've experienced. I went to the nurses and asked them to lock me in a side room. They just told me to go and sit down and watch the television. I kept going back to the office and in the end they gave me some tablets.

Another time I had a bad reaction to the injections I was having. I couldn't keep still. It was terrible, they said I was putting it on. That's the worst thing of all, not having your experience taken seriously.

Factors that help facilitate user self-empowerment

Some general points:

- Allow more time for people: for listening; for talking; for doing things together.
- Normalize the helping relationship.
- Avoid mystifying, excluding jargon.
- Respect the way people experience their reality.
- Respect the expertise of people in knowing what helps.
- Provide accessible information that people need to make informed choices and ensure it is understood.
- Encourage people to take a leading role in the care planning process, such as carrying out a self-assessment or introducing client-held records.
- Enable access to resources outside the service provision in meeting needs, such as adult education, recreational facilities, complementary therapies and counselling.
- Respect people's right to choose.
- Practise judicious non-intervention.
- Respect the client's right to the dignity of risk.
- Avoid coercion and threats.
- Celebrate people's achievements, successes, strengths and abilities.
- Nurture hopefulness.
- Help people gain the skills they need to feel more empowered and be more assertive.
- Acknowledge the impact of social inequalities and impoverishment on the lives of people who use the mental health services.
- Acknowledge the impact of stigma on the lives of people who use the mental health services.
- Openly discuss experiences of compulsory supervision, admission, detention and treatment.
- Encourage the use of independent advocacy.
- Encourage involvement in user groups and patient councils.
- Seek users' views on the service and encourage user-led research.
- Avoid pathologizing labels and deterministic explanations.

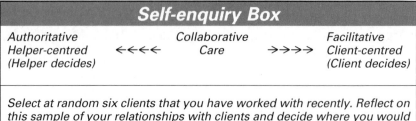

Authoritative		Collaborative		Facilitative
Helper-centred	←←←←	Care	→→→→	Client-centred
(Helper decides)				(Client decides)

Select at random six clients that you have worked with recently. Reflect on this sample of your relationships with clients and decide where you would put these along the continuum. Evaluate your response. What does it say about your approach to helping relationships? About your needs? About the client's way of relating to others? About the client's needs? What would you need to do to make your way of relating more client-centred and facilitative?

10 Advocacy and the working alliance

The United Kingdom Central Council for Nursing and Midwifery (UKCC) recognizes advocacy as an important element in mental health nursing. In their Guidelines for Mental Health and Disability Nursing (1998) they state:

> When caring for clients you must endeavour to promote and safeguard their interests. You must not practise in a way which assumes that only you know what's best for the client. This may create dependency, hinder teamwork and can interfere with the client's right to choose. Some clients may be highly suggestible and thus more likely to agree to suggestions or choices of those in positions of authority. Advocacy is about promoting clients' right to choose and empowering them to decide for themselves (p. 14).

While many nurses do speak out on behalf of clients often at some risk to their own position, there are difficulties associated with nurse advocacy. As the mental health nursing review team concluded in their report 'Working in Partnership' (Department of Health, 1994) 'because nurses are part of the service there is a potential for conflict of interest with their role as employees, their duty of care and professional ethics' (2.1.7).

The user movement too, has voiced reservations about nurses' ability to be true advocates and identifies conflict of interest, a lack of time and a lack of trust as being limiting factors. As Campbell (1996) puts it, 'There is always at some level a sense of a legal background to the relationship between users and mental health professionals – that treatment and hospitalization can be forced.'

There does now appear to be a shift away from nurses acting as advocates towards nurses working with advocates, as independent advocacy becomes more widely available. Independent advocates are people who are not employed by the service and who may or may not be users or ex-users of mental health services themselves. Usually they work as part of a co-ordinated local advocacy network. The independence of advocates is no guarantee that the relationship will be an empowering one and it is therefore important that self-advocacy is at the centre of advocacy practice. Given the right information, advice and encouragement, many clients are able to speak and act for themselves.

Working with users and their advocates is a new and challenging development in mental health care practice. At its best, it can enable clients to get the care and services they need and improve outcomes. It is essential that nurses inform themselves about local advocacy schemes and encourage the use of advocates. Working alongside users and their advocates requires an ability to negotiate so as to arrive at a position where clients' expressed needs and choices as well as their assessed needs, which may not always be the same, are being substantially met in a programme of care. It can sometimes be difficult for professionals to be open to advocacy, which in articulating clients' wishes might challenge what staff see as being in the best interest of the client. Advocacy confronts mental health professionals' often deeply held belief that all knowledge and expertise relevant to client care resides with them. For nurses, who have traditionally seen themselves as representing patients' needs and choices to other professionals and services, independent advocacy can seem to question the adequacy of this aspect of their role and diminish or threaten their special relationship with service users. These issues can lead to some tension and conflict in the relationship between nurses and advocates. Hopefully, as advocates become more familiar in the working environment, nurses will begin to rethink the boundaries of their responsibilities and any conflict that does arise will be used creatively to produce more effective care and better services. After all, both mental health nurses and independent advocates are working towards the same end, which is to facilitate self-advocacy and empowerment.

Jim' story *(Theme: the value of independent advocacy)*
Jim has been admitted to his local mental health unit following a psychiatric crisis. This is his fourth admission over the past 9 years. Jim's distressed disturbed behaviour takes the form of hearing voices, which accuse him of being responsible for criminal acts of a violent and sexual nature. He believes that he has no protection from evil forces at work in the world and relates this to an experience of being sexually abused by the leader of a church youth club. Jim's mood at these times is anxious, angry and despairing, most of which he holds in his rigidly tense musculature. He has been attending a local user-led group, which has helped strengthen his self-esteem and sense of being in control of his life.

Jim is aware that an increase in his medication is beneficial, as is having people to talk to. Being in hospital provides a safe environment in which he feels 'held' and this helps him deal with his chaotic inner world. He also knows that being able to take vigorous walks in the fresh air reduces the tension which seems to accumulate in his body and which has led to outbursts of destructive behaviour in the past.

Jim has now been in hospital for a couple of days. The current staff on the unit do not know Jim very well and his preferred strategies for managing crises are not clearly documented in his notes. Jim's primary nurse is working under some pressure owing to staff sickness and has not been able to respond sufficiently to his need to talk. With no outlet for his accumulating tension, Jim smashes a coffee table against a wall and has to be physically held. His medication is immediately increased. Over the next few days Jim com-

> plains of persistent drowsiness and begins to experience side effects. He finds it difficult to be assertive in asking for a reduction in his medication or for the care he needs. His fantasy is that the nurses and doctors will no longer take care of him and that he will be sent to prison.
>
> Jim's advocate, Max, visits him, and together they are able to review the incident and his care plan with his primary nurse.

Independent advocacy can be particularly helpful for clients whose experience is one of being discounted, disbelieved, devalued and discriminated against, as is the case for many people with long-term mental health problems. This is particularly true of black and other minority ethnic groups who find it difficult to get access to preferred treatments and facilities. An advocate from the client's own ethnic group can be invaluable in helping the client articulate the cultural differences that have implications for how psychosocial distress should be understood and managed.

In Advocacy – a Code of Practice (Conlon *et al.*, 1996) the User Group Task Force identify a number of situations in which independent advocacy can have a useful presence. These include:

- Crisis episodes. Some clients now carry crisis cards, which may include the name of their advocate as a person they wish to be contacted.
- Care programming meetings where an advocate may speak on behalf of the client or be a supportive presence.
- Where changes in treatment are being proposed, e.g. a new drug prescribed.
- Where a client is consulting a GP or psychiatrist about reducing or withdrawing from medication and needs support in having that choice respected.
- Changes in status under the Mental Health Act and appeals to a mental health tribunal.
- Supporting clients in carrying out a self-assessment.
- Supporting clients in developing their care plan with a key worker or primary nurse.
- Supporting clients in seeking to resolve issues involving benefits, housing, employment and transport.
- Helping clients to formalize complaints.
- Speaking on behalf of clients where there are language barriers and ethnicity issues.

Group advocacy in the form of user groups and patients councils has been slow to develop in the UK, although there are now several well developed groups in place – the United Kingdom Advocacy Network and Survivors Speak Out – which give the user movement an influential voice both locally and nationally. A number of user-led research projects have been published which offer valuable insights into the effectiveness of current services and identify areas of concern (Beeforth *et al.*, 1994; Mental Health Foundation, 1997; Rose *et al.*, 1998). There is an obligation on service providers to encourage the establishment of patient councils and to be open and responsive to feedback and complaints about the adequacy of the service. Patients may find it difficult to become involved and it is important that mental health professionals encourage and enable clients to do this by providing information about local groups and helping people acquire the skills they need to be participating members of such groups. As with individual advocacy, there is, for some professionals, a suspicion that group advocacy will necessarily be adversarial, led by the most vociferous users who may have a personal axe to grind and whose views are unrepresentative. Experience has mostly shown that these fears are unfounded and that where practitioners and management do not retreat into defensiveness and open discussion and collaboration take place, what results is a creative alliance that is to the benefit of all.

It is only through advocacy that the stigma and barriers to the integration of people with severe and long-term mental illness into the wider community will begin to be lifted. It requires people to come together – users, ex-users, carers, mental health professionals and citizens – in forums where a real understanding of the experience of people who experience severe psychological distress can take place. Perhaps then we shall see a service begin to evolve that is demystified, deprofessionalized and one which offers real community care.

Case management and the working alliance

Potentially, one of the most helpful strategies to come out of the Care in the Community Act (1990) is the requirement that people experiencing severe, long-term mental health problems should have a case manager. Onyett (1998) describes case management as a way of tailoring help to meet an individual's needs through placing responsibility for assessment and service co-ordination with one worker, who may also have a primary therapeutic role, function as an advocate, or act as a broker purchasing services on behalf of the client. In practice, there seems to be an axis along which case managers work, at one end of which their work is mainly concerned with coordinating the care provided by a number of agencies and, at the other, with intensive direct work with the client.

The case management role is clearly a challenging one, requiring considerable skill, knowledge and personal resources. Drawing on the literature, Onyett identifies a number of attributes necessary for workers to be effective. Case managers need to have experience of working with people experiencing severe, long-term mental health problems, be familiar with pharmacological and psychological interventions and have an awareness of community resources. In addition, they need to be able to offer families psychoeducational support and be aware of the impact of social disadvantage and discrimination on the lives of users. Studies during the early 1990s raised concerns that these skills might be lacking in community mental health teams, partly as the result of nurses developing caseloads that were over-represented with clients having short-term problems which were more responsive to psychotherapeutic interventions (Gournay, 1996). A number of influential reports since (Working in Partnership, Department of Health, 1994) have identified the needs of people with more severe and long-term problems as the 'proper focus' for mental health nursing and the profession is now redefining itself in relation to this client group.

Case management has its origins in the development of community mental health programmes in America in the 1980s. A number of these projects have provided the evidence base for the development of community services involving case management in the UK (see Onyett pp 37–70). A study of community mental health services in Madison County, which involved a highly vulnerable, socially disconnected group of people, with a diagnosis of schizophrenia and an average of five previous admissions, has been particularly influential. Key outcomes of this study showed a significantly reduced readmission rate compared with a control group receiving traditional psychiatric follow-up, as well as improved social functioning on a number of measures. After 12 months the community support programme was discontinued. Gains made under case management were soon lost as clients returned to traditional follow-up care. This finding is clearly important in highlighting the need for case management to be seen as a long-term service commitment to clients. Other features to emerge from this study were the importance of actively reaching out to clients, not allowing them to drop through the service net – an approach now referred to as assertive outreach. Also important was the accessibility of the service to clients and carers, 24 hours a day, seven days a week.

Overall case management seems to be valued by users and their families. One user-led study (Beeforth *et al.*, 1994) identifies the following experiences of case management as being important sources of user satisfaction:

- Greater client involvement in care planning.
- Access to appropriate services.
- Advice and practical help.
- Improvement in the quality of life.
- Family support.
- The on-going relationship with a case manager.

Case management is a rather inelegant term which suggests that people are seen as 'cases' to be 'managed' in a rather depersonalized, controlling way. In reality, as Beeforth's study suggests, case management can be highly person centred and empowering. Essential to its success is the relationship that develops between case manager and the person receiving care. A study by Repper *et al.* (1994) of relationships between case managers and their clients, identifies a number of values that seem important to this process. First, case managers need to recognize the slow pace of change and take a long-term view. Maintaining an attitude of realistic hopefulness helps them and their clients avoid a sense of frustration and failure. As the well-known Chinese proverb puts it 'a journey of a thousand miles begins with a single step'. Second, the ability of case managers to develop an empathic understanding of the client's experience is vital to building a trusting relationship. The chaos that manifests itself in the outer world of highly vulnerable people can reflect the chaos in their inner world. Case managers need the intuitive ability to enter that world without losing a foothold in their own. Being deeply understood in this way helps connect clients with another, so that they are no longer adrift in the uncharted oceans of their own consciousness. Finally, case managers need to be flexible in their approach to working with clients. A service that listens and is responsive to the expressed needs of clients as individuals is valued. Avoiding a tendency to fit people into existing services and systems, whether they want it or not and whether it is likely to meet their needs or not, can lead to creative collaboration in care planning. Some users may not want regular contact with the case manager or will only accept brief informal contact. In the work with some clients, there will be what Onyett calls 'episodic closure' during periods of well-being. The important issue here is that access to the service should be kept open and that carers, general practitioners, primary care staff and others in the client's

me you've been abused all your life Dawn – she's right I have. I get really depressed sometimes and I get this idea in my head that I'm sort of responsible for all the bad things that happen.

Irene's story (case manager)

I've been working with Dawn for about $2\frac{1}{2}$ years now. We didn't really have a relationship for a long while. She didn't want anything to do with the mental health services and was quite resentful and at times verbally abusive towards me. She would never let me into her flat. I was really only able to engage with her through Rolly, her boyfriend. The breakthrough came when he became ill and died. I was able to help her through his death, practically and emotionally. I don't think she had experienced someone just being there for her before. Most of her life she's experienced abuse and abandonment. In a way that's been replicated by the way health and social services have treated her over the years. She's had all sorts of people involved in her care at one time or another. To have a consistent relationship with one person has helped her a lot. I think she trusts me now, although she still tests me out from time to time – being unpleasant or unresponsive to me to see if I care about her enough. I have had to be quite careful with my boundaries. At one time she became very curious about my personal life and was quite possessive and demanding making out she was a lot worse than she was.

When she started being more open with me about her problems, she let me into her flat. It was very chaotic, not at all homely. It made me realize that home is a concept that doesn't really mean much to her. One of the things we've been working together is home making as well as her home management skills. At the moment I'm going in three times a week. She's going through an unsettled phase again. I think it's partly that Christmas is getting close, which is always a bad time for her, but also it's the anniversary of Rolly's death. She's also having a bit of hassle with the housing department who she feels want her out. Apparently she's been putting rubbish down the toilet and sink rather than using the dustbin. The problem was that a neighbour had told her off for using the wrong bin. There has been a bit of prejudice toward her in the flats, which is one of the reasons why she didn't want me calling round initially.

If Dawn feels rejected she starts cutting herself or smashing things, her arms are road maps of scar tissue. The worst thing is that she feels bad and that she deserves to be neglected and abused. There have been times in the past when she's gone out and picked men up and had casual sex with them, partly because of her need for human contact and partly because she has little respect for herself. The group has helped her a lot with her self-esteem. I think she felt that she felt able to give something of value to others, which is a new experience for Dawn. It was important the group was a positive experience because it could open the door to other resources that she's refused to consider in the past.

I know she hates the thought of having to go back into hospital. Dawn's behaviour has been quite challenging in the past and she has found the care oppressive. I've tried to be open with her about what I would and wouldn't do.

12

The working alliance with families and carers

The success of community-orientated psychiatry depends on a real partnership being forged between informal carers and mental health professionals. The National Service Framework for Mental Health (Department of Health, 1999) identifies caring for carers as central to the task of improving standards of mental health care. It acknowledges that carers play a vital role in helping to look after users of the mental health services, particularly those with long-term mental health problems. Between 50 and 70% of people who have been diagnosed as suffering from schizophrenia live with their families (Marks *et al.*, 1994). The framework recognizes the strains and responsibilities of caring, as well as the satisfactions, and acknowledges the impact it can have on carers' mental and physical health. It sets out the standards to be achieved by local mental health services in relation to caring for carers, which includes an assessment of needs and the formulation of a care plan for carers. For a real partnership to develop, both sides must recognize and accept the expertise of the other and the advantages and disadvantages of the formal professional role and the role of informal carer.

A guide for action produced by The King's Fund (Richardson, 1989) has yet to be fully or universally implemented. Its recommendations will need to be substantially adopted if the strategic framework for improving standards in mental health services is to be successful.

Carers need:

- Recognition of their contribution and of their own needs as individuals in their own right.
- Services tailored to individual circumstances, needs and views, through discussion at the time help is being planned.
- Services that reflect and are sensitive to, the differing racial, cultural and religious backgrounds of families and are equally accessible to carers of every race and ethnic origin.
- Opportunities for a break, both for short spells (an afternoon) and for longer periods (a week or more), to relax and to have time to themselves.
- Practical help to lighten the tasks of caring.
- Someone to talk to about their emotional needs, at the outset of caring, while they are caring and when the caring task is over.
- Information about available benefits and services.

- Information about a family member's vulnerability/disability and treatment and how to cope with problematic behaviour.
- Opportunities to explore alternatives to family care both in the immediate and long-term future.
- Services developed through consultation with carers at all levels of the organization.

Not only are carers and families facing the emotional strain of living with a person whose behaviour is problematic, they may also be experiencing the pangs of grief. Enduring and disabling mental illness constitutes a loss for the family. It can seem as if the person being cared for has become trapped and unreachable in their troubled, perplexing world. Hopes and aspirations begin to recede, as the long-term nature of the disability becomes apparent. Families need time and help to accept the reality of the disability and the implications and meanings it has for them. They need time to acknowledge the pain of the loss and work through the feelings that may recur over many months, perhaps even years. As the grieving process unfolds, help may be needed to adjust to the change in their lives and to find constructive ways of living with a family member who has an enduring vulnerability and disability. Finally, carers and families may need encouragement and support to invest emotional energy, not just in the provision of continuing care, but in other relationships, both inside and outside the family, and in living their own lives.

Much of the research on families has investigated the family as a factor in causation and as an influence on outcome in major mental health problems. The hardship and burden of living with a severely troubled family member is well recognized, although its impact on carers and the family system has not been extensively researched. The studies that there have been, suggest that up to one-third of carers suffers from depression and anxiety (Fadden *et al.,* 1987). Neither has the positive influence of the family been fully recognized. Professional workers seldom assess a family's strengths as a resource for increasing and maintaining the well-being of family members.

Families are not always easy to engage. Intervention studies report that up to 35% of families refuse therapeutic help and up to 50% withdraw from intervention programmes (Barrowclough and Tarrier, 1997). Follow-up studies of this non-engaged group show a higher relapse rate. A number of factors appear influential in determining whether a family participates in an intervention programme. Some families may have a negative perception of the mental health services based on previous experience. They may have been made to feel as if their experience and knowledge of a person's vulnerability and disability over many years counts for nothing. There may be a sense of resignation and hopelessness about the future; the feeling that whatever is done will make no appreciable difference. Often there is a defensiveness towards mental health professionals arising out of a fear of blame that creates a barrier to engagement. It is not uncommon for families to close up protectively, locating the problem firmly within the individual, and to resist any attempt to attribute it to difficulties within the family system.

Over the last 30 years there has been a strong research interest in the link between relapse patterns and stress within the family system. Living and coping with a relative who experiences disruptive changes in mood, or becomes apathetic, withdrawn and reclusive, or is troubled by voice hearing and unusual beliefs, can create enormous tension. In families where high levels of hostility and criticism occur in response to problematic behaviour or where care is given in an over intrusive, over involved way – an interaction pattern referred to as 'high expressed emotion' – recurrence of the disruptive distress is likely to occur. This is linked with the stress-vulnerability theory of schizophrenia which argues that certain individuals have a neuropathology that predisposes them to distress patterns likely to be labelled psychotic when faced with stressful social situations, particularly if their coping strategies are poorly developed.

Several family intervention studies involving 'high expressed emotion' families have shown that it is possible to improve relapse rates and improve the social functioning of clients (Leff *et al.*, 1982, 1985; Tarrier *et al.*, 1988, 1989). Kuipers (1991) suggests that family intervention should aim to:

- Reduce family criticism and increase tolerance of problems.
- Reduce relatives' over involvement and encourage the client's independence.
- Engage the family in a creative problem-solving process to manage problematic behaviour.
- Defuse emotional tension and encourage a sense of realistic optimism.
- Improve the client's coping skills and social functioning.

These needs may be met in the context of a psycho-educational programme that offers education about the illness, stress management, problem-solving and goal-setting. Barrowclough and Tarrier suggest that an intervention that seeks to change family interaction patterns will need to be seen as a long- term engagement of 12 months or more. Programmes that aim primarily to provide information and support to groups of families and carers are usually of shorter duration. Atkinson and Cola (1995) suggest ten sessions over a period of 20 weeks.

Reducing negativity

Some aspects of a client's distressed behaviour can generate strong feelings in family members. There may be high levels of irritation, annoyance, resentment and hostility in the family environment. Often intolerance is linked with ineffective coping and negative attributions associated with the problem behaviour. For example, apathy and inertia may be seen as laziness and perversity. Preoccupation with unusual ideas or behaving in unusual ways may be seen as foolishness. Sharing information about the nature of a person's vulnerability and disability and their treatment and care aims to increase tolerance and reduce criticism. Families, it is hoped, are then able to develop a more informed perspective on the problem behaviour and hold more realistic expectations.

In reviewing studies of the effectiveness of brief education, Barrowclough and Tarrier conclude that it is worthwhile, in that it increases relatives' knowledge of the disability and improves the well-being of carers, at least in the short term. It can also 'prepare relatives for changing their behaviour' in response to longer-term family intervention. However, brief education by itself seems to have little effect on the way carers and families cope with problem behaviour or on the outcome of the client's vulnerability. They argue that education is best started early in the course of the disability, before a family's personal explanatory theories and strategies for coping have had time to become established. Where a relative's disability has existed for some time, education needs to be seen as long term and part of the total family intervention package. Education is best approached in an involving way. While a practitioner's educational input can be structured around relevant themes and given in conjunction with information booklets, relatives need the opportunity to discuss their own understandings, anxieties, practical difficulties and their adopted solutions.

Reducing oversolicitous care

Overinvolvement is a term used to describe the kind of relationship in which there is an inappropriate level of dependence and over-protectiveness. It is most often seen, although not exclusively, as a feature of the relationship between a parental carer and an adult son or daughter who has an enduring mental health problem. Although troubled individuals may require considerable assistance in dealing with the challenges and opportunities of everyday living, too much care can hold people in a dependent state and block the recovery process. Often dependent relationships pre-date the emergence of the disability and reflect the emotional needs of the carer and the organization of the family system. The task of the professional may be to enter the family system in a way that allows some realignment of roles and relationships to take place. Bringing about some change in the relationship can be a lengthy process and finding the right lever is important. It can be helpful to emphasize the client's adulthood and the need for appropriate age-related functioning. It can be helpful to discuss the need for positive risk-taking and the low probability of the carer's worst fears being realized. Emphasizing the carer's need for an independent life and, as it were, 'giving permission' for this to happen, can initiate change. Sometimes an acknowledgement of the fact that the carer will not be able to fulfil that role forever can lead to a recognition of the importance of the client preparing for a more independent life style.

Limit setting can be difficult for carers, but is essential if they are not to be exploited and abused. Often demanding or aggressive behaviour has become an established pattern and relatives may go on suffering this unreasonable behaviour because a person is 'ill'. It is important that carers are helped to see that the person they are caring for is able to take adult responsibility for their behaviour despite their disability. Limits should be negotiated with the person being cared for that recognize the carer's rights and needs and these should be held to consistently. It can be very difficult to persuade clients with overinvolved relationships to engage in a planned programme aimed at strengthening their life skills and building their confidence and independence. Some of the worries that exist around separation and individuation for the carer and client may have to be addressed first, otherwise attempts to help the client move towards more independent living will be blocked.

Creative problem management

Successful family intervention involves engaging families in collaborative problem solving. This can be helpful not only in changing their response to problematic behaviour, but also in dissolving some of the hopelessness and resignation that may have built up over years of unsupported caring. Engaging families in problem solving may not be easy. Kuipers comments that some resistance from relatives may derive from them seeing an implicit criticism in the mental health professional's optimism. The possibility that some difficult aspect of a client's behaviour is reducible by dealing with it differently or applying a strategy more persistently or consistently, may imply that they have not been making enough effort. It is important for carers and relatives not to feel the problem behaviour is being minimized or their way of coping over the years is seen as 'wrong'. Behaviour that carers and families may find difficult and distressing typically includes apathy and inertia, withdrawal from the world outside and within the family, excessive dependency, aggressiveness, odd behaviour, voice hearing and the presence of disturbing delusional ideas in the client's conversation. It is also important to keep in mind that suicide has an increased incidence in seriously troubled people with enduring problems and families may be burdened by worries about the safety of the person they are caring for. The problem behaviour should be identified as specifically as possible. Problems which are most pressing, which are amenable to change and can be worked on, should be given priority. Often desired outcomes can be broken down into smaller achievable goals, each of which represents a tangible improvement in the situation. You may find it helpful to revisit the framework for managing problems discussed earlier in this part of the book.

Simon's story *(Theme: family work in enduring mental health problems)*
Simon is a 32-year-old man who became extremely troubled when he was seventeen and was subsequently diagnosed as suffering from schizophrenia. He has remained very vulnerable to episodes of disabling distress, during which he is disturbed by troubling thoughts and accusatory voices. Over the past 15 years he has been admitted to the local psychiatric unit on nine occasions. Many of his admission experiences have been distressing events, which have left Simon feeling very wary of the psychiatric services. He often says that he feels diminished and degraded by his psychiatric status and, as a consequence, will sometimes deny his continuing vulnerability, refuse medication and express a reluctance to have any further contact with mental health professionals. There are times when he is depressed and discouraged by the emptiness of his life and at these times he will often ask his GP for 'euthanasia', which is indicative of the hopelessness and despair he feels.

There have been attempts to accommodate Simon in supported housing, but his tenancy has broken down owing to his refusal of support and his threatening behaviour towards fellow tenants and project staff. He lived in a hostel for the homeless for a while but, for the past 7 years, has lived at home with his mother and step-father. He has two married stepsisters – one lives locally, the other abroad. His own father committed suicide when Simon was four. While his mother and stepfather have a sense of duty towards their son and are deeply concerned for him, the burden of having him live with them has been considerable and has undermined the warmth of their affection for him. Simon is a chaotic presence in their lives, which have become disrupted and strained. His step-father gets angry at what he sees as Simon's 'nonsense' and 'lazi-ness' and feels he could 'make more of an effort'. Simon's mother, who is his main carer, has an appeasing attitude towards him and finds it difficult to set limits. She carries a sense of guilt about Simon's problems and blames herself when he refuses medication and 'sacks' mental health staff involved in his care. Both his par-ents find it very difficult to deal with his persecutory, deluded think-ing that emerges at times of stress and his demanding and apathetic behaviour has 'defeated' them. Simon's presence in the house has made it difficult for his parents to have a social life, to go out and leave him, or to invite people in. His mother has become particularly isolated in her role as Simon's carer and is currently taking antidepressants.

Despite the somewhat gloomy overview there is a continuing desire to help Simon to move forward in his life. Simon himself recognizes that he should have 'spread his wings' by now, but enjoys the comfort of home and the company, feeling that he would be quite lonely if he lived by himself.

Family intervention

The family: Simon, his parents and his stepsister were seen as a group and at other times the parents were seen alone. It was explained that caring for people like Simon, with a vulnerability to troubled states of mind, can be stressful and burdensome for all families and that sometimes the stress that builds up can ag-gravate the disorder. Therefore, it made sense to look at ways of trying to reduce the difficulties and the amount of stress the family experienced. The family was invited to meet with the family worker and co-worker over a period of about a year, first at weekly inter-vals, then monthly. This was accepted readily by the parents. Simon was reluctant to agree, but had no objection to his parents attending the meetings.

The first two sessions were attended by the parents and sister and were spent talking about the nature of Simon's vulnerability. Because the term schizophrenia can be such a frightening label to many people and has such a pervasive impact on identity, it was not a term that was used. Instead the stress vulnerability model was explained indicating that for some people the stress reaction could be quite extreme and disabling, as in Simon's case. It seemed important to release Simon from the power of the label and emphasize that the problem is the problem not the person! Like anyone else Simon had faults and failings, but also strengths, abilities, hopes and aspirations that can easily become obscured by disabilities. The family was invited to identify some attributes or characteristics that they valued and appreciated about each other before the next meeting. The intention was to help the family reconnect with some of the more positive feelings they felt towards Simon. This brought up more than liked characteristics, setting off a discussion on Simon's abilities and interests, past and present. The fact that he used to swim for a swimming club, that he is interested in classic cars, that he likes and is good with dogs, that he is knowledgeable about films. In the wake of this discussion, feelings of sadness, anguish and bitterness about the loss of the life not lived began to emerge. His mother spoke about feeling in some way to blame for his affliction and acknowledged that she 'did too much for him' and 'gave in to him' too often to mitigate this guilt. She also talked about her anger and guilt at the time of her first husband's death and the fear that the same thing would happen to Simon. Simon's stepfather talked about how he had never felt able to act as an authoritative parent. It was agreed that the family worker should write to Simon bringing him up to date with what had been talked about so far and inviting him to the next meeting.

An early focus in the work was to look at how 'the trouble', as it came to be called, had a grip on their lives and on Simon's life. They were asked to describe how 'the trouble' got them down, how it interfered with life, how it caused them to react. Following on from this they were asked about the ways in which they were able to influence 'the trouble'. The task set for them was to notice how they loosened its grip on their lives so that it wasn't so restricting, upsetting and difficult. How they reacted to 'the trouble', what they said or did that made a difference. This yielded some useful strategies that both the family and Simon were already using to cope with difficult behaviour. These coping strategies were reinforced and other suggestions made about what they might try. One aspect of this was emphasizing reasonableness of setting limits and the right to a life of their own. A key part of this discussion centred on re-evaluating the parent's fears about what would happen if Simon was at home alone and the need for positive risk-taking.

Finding a way of enabling Simon to become more independent proved difficult. Although he agreed that at his age he should be 'in charge of his life', he did not show any inclination to take responsibility for managing it. There was some discussion with the parents about their own experiences of growing towards independence and they both reflected that leaving home and 'having to look after yourself because there was no one else to do it for you' was the spur. Some realistic self-care goals were agreed, the parents recognizing that Simon needed a similar spur in order to become more resourceful and autonomous.

> A particularly significant event took place in one session when Joanna (Simon's stepsister) talked about a time when she had been involved in an accident and had to spend weeks in bed recovering. She described how her 'big brother' had spent a lot of time with her and made her laugh at a time when she was in discomfort and upset. The whole family then engaged in some enjoyable reverie about 'Simon the joker', an aspect of his personality that had become submerged beneath the dark pools of distress that had flooded his mind since his late teens. This created an opportunity to strengthen the sibling bond and led to Joanna becoming a more active and supportive presence in Simon's life.
>
> The work continued for 18 months. During that time the emotional tension that had been a constant feature of family life eased and Simon's troubled chaotic behaviour diminished.

Reducing the emotional labour of caring

Caring for a person with an enduring mental health problem is an emotional labour. Members of the family may experience a wide range of powerful and upsetting emotions. As discussed above, these may be associated with the experience of grief. In addition, many parents experience feelings of guilt, thinking that they are in some way to blame for the problem. There may be intense feelings of irritation, resentment and anger at the demands and difficulties posed by the client's behaviour. Fearfulness about the risks posed by a relative's behaviour and anxiety about the possibility of relapse are also commonly experienced. There is also the additional burden of living with the stigma of long-term mental health problems and the isolation that may cause. There may be frustration and disillusionment with the mental health services because of lack of consultation and support, or the lack of continuity owing to frequent staff changes. The failure of psychiatry to cure the problem adds to a sense of disillusionment and despondency. High levels of distress over a long period can cause carers to burn out and no longer be able to provide care conducive to recovery. Sometimes, a family unable to cope any longer with the stress of continuing care may reject the client.

Helping carers and the family manage their distress is an important component of family-centred care. It is important not only from the point of view of the well-being of carers and other family members, but also a high degree of emotional tension in the family environment may lead to a greater likelihood of relapse occurring. Barrowclough and Tarrier outline the rationale for stress management in the following way:

- Living with a person who suffers from schizophrenia can be very difficult and it is usual for relatives to feel stressed or upset at least some of the time.
- When a patient is living with the family, a lot of the day-to-day help and rehabilitation is carried out by family members. Hence it is important to make sure they, in turn, have help in managing their own feelings in

coping with difficult situations if they are to go on helping the patient effectively.

- People who suffer from schizophrenia are unusually sensitive to the stress of others; therefore by feeling more in control of themselves relatives are indirectly helping the patient.

Care should be taken in making this last point to families as it can easily be heard as blame. The positives of stress management should be emphasized rather than the negative consequences for the client of the carers' stress.

Reducing the family's experience of distress can have a twin focus. First, if other more effective ways of responding to difficult behaviour can be found, or if that behaviour can be modified by some other intervention, for example by a change in medication or by helping the client develop a more effective coping strategy, then their distress levels should be reduced. Second, carers and others in the family can be taught how to manage their stress levels in a way that prevents the build-up of distress and exhaustion. It is important for professionals to accept and contain the ventilation of feelings and to normalize these feelings, particularly the negative ones, emphasizing that they would be expected in any family faced with experience of caring for a relative who has become deeply troubled. A useful strategy when working with negative feelings is reframing (Kuipers *et al.*, 1992). It is usually possible to point out the positives in the painful feelings that surface in families. Underneath the angry accusation 'you do nothing but sit around all day' is a real concern about a son or daughter losing out on life. 'I wish you'd stop behaving so stupidly, we'd get on a lot better' can be reframed as, 'Much as I want to, it's difficult for me to feel close to you and be around you when you behave in that way.' Talking about feelings, either on an individual basis or in the family group, can help reduce tension and discord. When the person being cared for is present, it is important that the emotions expressed are linked with specific behaviours and not seen as a rejection of the whole person. 'I can't trust you any more', is better expressed as, 'When you wander around the house at night and leave the fire and the grill on, it leaves me feeling I can't rely on you.' Where relatives' groups exist, they can offer a useful forum for sharing feelings in an atmosphere of mutuality. The fact that other people have experienced the same distress reduces carers' worries about the unreasonableness of their feelings and offers ways of coping more effectively.

It can be useful to ask family members to keep a journal of situations that arise which result in them becoming emotionally upset. Self-monitoring requires relatives to record the situation, how they felt, what they thought and what they did. Barrowclough and Tarrier emphasize the need for interventions that aim to help carers and families to manage stress in response to their specific experience rather than in the form of generalized techniques and strategies. This approach to managing stress involves three possibilities. First, the family and practitioner can look at the situation that the carers find distressing and consider ways of changing it. That might involve changing the client's behaviour or changing the relatives' behavioural response to it. Second, it could involve changing the way the situation is perceived: often the distress people experience arises not so much from the situation itself as from the way they see it. Thinking errors may be present, for example, anxiety about going out and leaving someone in the house alone may be based on unreasonable fears about what might happen. Finally, people can learn to change the way they react internally through learning relaxation techniques, having periods of respite, removing themselves from situations that trigger distress, comforting themselves and building 'comfort zones' that offer an oasis of calm in their life.

Enhancing coping and social functioning

While family interventions are aimed at the family system, the approach we are discussing here also focuses more directly on improving the social functioning of the vulnerable family member. This allows others in the family to become involved in helping to develop constructive behaviour. Any positive change in the client's behaviour can promote a feeling of hopefulness and reduce the sense of burden and stress experienced by the family. Barrowclough and Tarrier suggest an approach that aims to build up constructive behaviour through goal setting. A helpful starting point in this process is for the client and family to identify strengths, which can later be drawn on in setting goals and action planning. Strengths may include interests, abilities, talents, personal qualities, aspirations and resources. For example, a client's paranoid anxiety and reclusive lifestyle was reduced by exploiting his interest in films and sport to create opportunities to pursue those interests in ways that involved an increasing level of 'safe contact' with others.

Problems and difficulties that are identified by carers, the family and the client in the present scenario can lead to a discussion about the preferred scenario, out of which achievable goals emerge. Asking the client and the family future-orientated questions such as, 'If a spontaneous improvement were to take place and things were 10% better than they are now, what would you notice that would be different?' or, 'What needs to be different for you to feel better about this situation?' Once clear goals and desired outcomes have been established, strategies can be devised with the client and family to achieve them. Sometimes it can be helpful to ask about 'exceptions', times when the problematic behaviour has not occurred or occurred less, times when the preferred scenario has, if only partially and briefly, occurred. This more future-orientated, solution-focused, optimistic problem management approach counteracts gloomy, pessimistic, problem-saturated reviews of the family's experience. Rather than focusing too much on the problem of, for example, a client's apathy, inertia and social withdrawal, it is more helpful look at ways in which the client and the family can influence the problem. Can they begin to have some influence on this 'retreat from the world', this 'immobility', rather than the problem having such a dominating and adverse influence on their lives. Similarly, the problem of stigmatizing, disruptive verbalization in response to persistent voices can involve the client and the family in finding strategies for managing the voice hearing in more socially adaptive ways. You may find it useful to revisit the framework for managing problems discussed earlier in this part of the book.

Nick and Beth's story *(Theme: the impact of the carer's role on marital relationships)*
Nick and Beth are a couple in their early thirties who have been married for 8 years and have a daughter aged six and a son aged four. Beth became very troubled and distressed following her daughter's birth and was diagnosed as suffering from puerperal psychosis. Since then her vulnerability has continued to express itself in three further episodes of acute distress which have required a period of hospitalization. During these episodes she is troubled by somatic sensations and thoughts that her body is changing, she complains that she is not real or that she is no longer in her body. At these times she has inflicted injuries on herself to prove 'I'm still alive'.

Around the time of Beth's second breakdown Nick was made redundant from his job as a laboratory technician and decided to stay at home to bring up his children and become Beth's primary carer. They have considerable support from Beth's mother who provides respite for Nick by having Beth and the children to stay once a month.

Recently the family asked for help because Beth was showing early signs of another relapse. There has been continuing tension in their relationship, with frequent, sometimes violent, rows. Some of the tension centres around the way their respective roles have evolved. Nick has taken over most of the responsibility for managing the home and caring for the children leaving Beth with what she sees as a subsidiary role. Her conception of herself as a capable parent is further diminished by her mother who 'takes charge' of the children during respite weekends. Beth is feeling like a third child and resents it. She has found it quite difficult to express her frustration because of the powerful coalition between her husband and her mother and because she fears that Nick might leave her and that she then might lose the children altogether. She resents the fact that there is little of the tenderness, affection and playfulness he shows towards the children in his relationship with her.

Nick feels that Beth's talents have never been in running a home. He argues that she seldom does things properly and the house would be in chaos if he left it to her. From his perspective both he and his mother-in-law are trying to protect her from the demands of being responsible for two lively, 'difficult' children. He says Beth is often overly anxious about the children and has at times visited the school several times during the day to reassure herself that her daughter was alright. He gets angry with her over her preoccupied state of mind and her unusual beliefs, which appear when she is stressed. He is often frustrated by her lack of motivation and indolence. Nick feels guilty about his impatience, intolerance and loss of temper, he says 'I should be big enough to accept that Beth is different.' He recalls that one of the things that attracted him to her in the first place was her 'oddity' and dreaminess. He recently experienced a family bereavement and felt unable to share his feelings with Beth, which confronted him with the emptiness in their relationship and with his own loneliness.

The family intervention which, at various times, involved Nick and Beth together and separately and Beth's mother, continued weekly at first and then monthly over a period of a year. It centred on the task of strengthening the relationship between Nick and Beth by creating opportunities for them to have time for themselves and on building up Beth's parental role and her conception of herself as a capable parent. It emerged that Beth had been carrying a deep sense of guilt and resentment about not being able to care for her daughter in the early months of her life because of the onset of her psychosis. She had as a result never really felt that her daughter 'was hers' and worried that she may have 'damaged her' by not being a 'proper mum'. There was also some work with Nick around managing stress and dealing with the strong feelings that his caring role triggered. An important factor to emerge in relation to Nick's caring role was that he had grown up in a family in which his father had left his alcoholic mother when he was six. As he grew up he increasingly took on the responsibility of 'parenting' his mother. It seemed that a repetition of this earlier script was being played out in the relationship between Nick and Beth. It was helpful to Nick to relocate some of the intense feelings he was experiencing in the 'here and now' of his relationship with Beth back into their rightful place of the 'there and then' relationship with his mother.

While engaging and working with the whole family is the ideal, some clients are not willing to have their family involved. This raises a difficult ethical issue. Can a carer be seen as a co-worker with rights to information about the client and to be involved in care planning? Can carers and families be seen as co-clients with rights to professional help? In the model of care we have been discussing above, there are elements of both positions. Part of the difficulty lies in the changing family role, from the family as a natural source of care to the more designated role of 'primary carer'. This subtle shift can have significant implications for the relationship between marital partners where one is the carer or between a parent and an adult child and with any other permutation. It is not difficult to see how strategic interventions, or early signs monitoring might be resented, or how the loss of reciprocity of care between spouses, where one has a long-term mental health problem, could undermine the relationship.

Much of what we have been discussing above in relation to family carers could also be applied to carers in others settings. Elements of 'high expressed emotion' may be a feature of the interaction between staff and clients in residential and ward settings. Critical, negative perceptions of residents may develop and cynicism and therapeutic nihilism creep in. Overbearing, directive, oversolicitous care can become the norm in the culture of a staff group whose anxieties are not being heard and contained, so that it is difficult to allow residents the dignity of risk and to nurture self-determination and self-reliance. Staff face high levels of stress and can

Self-enquiry Box

A genogram is a graphic and succinct way of organizing family history.

The problems facing the referred family can be seen in the context of a wider family system. It can highlight patterns and themes that have recurred through successive generations and are influencing the present and can draw attention to significant events and transitions.

Nick and Beth's genogram is given below. What questions might the genogram prompt?

Complete a genogram for your own family. What patterns, themes, significant events and transitions are brought into relief? What arouses your curiosity?

Complete a genogram for a family you are currently working with.

Workaholic emotionally distant	*Suffers from alcoholism*	*Divorced and remarried*	

Ruth	*Beth*	*Nick*	*Owen*	*Janet*
Stillborn	*Age 32*	*Age 34*	*Age 50*	*Died in an R.T.A. 9 months ago Age 47*

Jonathan	*Victoria*
Age 4	*Age 6*
Started school	*Suffers from enuresis*

Figure 12.1 Nick and Beth's genogram

become seriously depleted, with a risk to their own well-being, in organizations where the emotional labour of providing therapeutic care is not openly acknowledged and mitigated through supportive, replenishing structures.

Reluctance, resistance and the working alliance

Maintaining a working alliance can be difficult when compliance issues arise. These may be around continuing medication, accepting on-going contact with a mental health worker, attending a mental health resource centre, or the need for admission as a consequence of risk behaviour. These issues are best confronted in an honest way, acknowledging and respecting the feelings and fears of the client, while emphasizing their needs and responsibilities. Some reluctance and non-compliance should be seen as a healthy response to professional interventions that may involve surrendering some sovereignty over one's life to others. Not adhering to a prescribed care plan may be indicative of the spirit of recovery. It is an expression of an individual's personal power, a willingness to take some responsibility for themselves and their lives to claim a different identity from the one 'assigned' to them by mental health professionals.

Public concerns about care in the community have centred on those with severe, enduring mental health problems, who are difficult for services to engage. It is estimated that there are approximately 15 000 people who come within this group (Sainsbury Centre, 1998a). They are a group of people with diverse problems. Many are homeless. Others engage in problematic drug or alcohol use. Some have a history of offending behaviour. This group includes people who represent a risk to others or to themselves through self-neglect or suicide and who require assertive, proactive care.

The Richie report (1994) identified that there are between 3000 and 4000 people nationally who represent a high risk and require intensive supervision in the community. Supervision registers were introduced the same year in response to this need, but have not proved a satisfactory solution to risk minimization. Homicides and suicides involving people with severe mental disorders have continued at the rate of 40 per year and 1000 per year respectively. Much of the debate about the supervision of reluctant service users who are at risk has centred on the ethics and practicalities of compulsory treatment orders which will come into effect under new mental health legislation. Morgan and Hemming (1999) argue that the proposed legislation is a step too far towards enforcement and control which is likely to drive people further away from the service. While medication may be an important element in a care and treatment package, it alone will not eliminate risk. Risk minimization is more likely to become a reality if there is a continuing engagement with service users based on a negotiated plan that reflects psycho-social needs and emphasizes the responsibilities of the service as much as adherence on the part of service users. The high profile public enquiries, which are a requirement following homicides involving a mentally-disordered offender, have inadvertently increased public anxiety about community care. There is a widely held perception that the severely mentally ill living in the community represent a danger to the public. In fact, while violent crime and homicide convictions have increased since the 1960s, the proportion committed by people with severe mental health problems has decreased during a period when the closure of mental hospitals has gathered momentum.

Why do some people find it particularly difficult to engage with the mental health service? The Sainsbury Centre Review highlights the following factors: often people will have had negative experience of statutory services. They may, for example, have been in care as a child, or had a child taken into care. Many have had frustrating experiences with the Department of Social Security and Housing Departments. They may have had bewildering and frightening experiences of the criminal justice system, perhaps at a time of psychiatric crisis. Their previous experiences of being in hospital may have been traumatizing and may include being compulsorily admitted under a section of the Mental Health Act or being subjected to control, restraint or seclusion, receiving enforced medication or experiencing unpleasant side effects. Little wonder that a legacy of distrust persists in some people with severe mental health problems and that they are unwilling to engage with the service.

A disproportionate number of people with severe and enduring mental illness in the UK come from ethnic minority backgrounds and are over-represented in the group of clients who do not readily engage with the mental health services (Fernando, 1995). This can be partly understood as a reaction to the covert racism that exists among mental health workers. While overt prejudice may be rare, many nurses are ill informed and insensitive to the cultural norms, religious beliefs and social experience of people from ethnic minority communities. Copsey (1997), in a study of the provision of mental health services within a multi-faith community in a London borough, makes a strong case for:

- Employing mental health workers who reflect the ethnic diversity of the community.
- Establishing an ongoing training programme in cultural and spiritual sensitivity.
- Engaging in an respectful dialogue with local faith communities in order to learn about this significant dimension of people's lives.
- Working with various community groups to encourage and support care by the community.

Establishing and maintaining an alliance with this client group requires considerable skill that is best channelled through assertive outreach or high support teams. There is some evidence that services such as these can be effective in building a working alliance with non-compliant clients who have severe and complex problems, helping them to achieve some order and stability in their lives (Marks *et al.*, 1994; Ford and Ryan, 1997). The

Sainsbury Centre Review identifies a number of attributes and approaches that seem helpful in establishing a working alliance:

- There needs to be a commitment to a long-term relationship, with realistic objectives established.
- Allowing the user's priorities to set the agenda. This often involves problems with housing or benefits. Practical help can lead to the building of a therapeutic bond.
- Nurses need to be able to accept some florid symptoms, focusing on establishing a bond and maintaining engagement in the early stages, before making more active psychiatric interventions.
- Nurses should be prepared to work in informal settings – the street, a café, a local park.
- Having a similar social or ethnic background to the person using the service can help. Insensitivity to, or ignorance of a client's culture and religious beliefs is highlighted by service users from ethnic minority communities as a continuing issue. Ex-service users can have a valued role in some assertive outreach teams.
- People with low expressed emotion seem to work particularly well with this client group.

Non-adherence to medication is a significant issue in the community care of people with severe or enduring mental health problems and particularly those who are reluctant to engage with the service. It is a central factor in relapse, deterioration in psychological and social functioning and an increased risk to self and others. Unpleasant side effects are given as one reason for stopping medication. Coming to terms with having a long-term illness that requires continuing medication is another. But there are other factors. Leete (1987) makes the important observation that medication is sometimes linked in the minds of users with power and control. Rejecting medication can be as much about rejecting authority and regaining some say over their lives, as denying the therapeutic benefits of medication. What is needed here is a trusting relationship with a key worker in which there is:

- Openness about medication, with information effectively given. A realistic expectation of medication is encouraged. Fears and feelings about medication are heard.
- Help with coming to terms with having a long-term psychiatric illness that requires long-term medication.
- Advocacy and support for a client wishing to try different neuroleptic medication, in order to find one that causes minimum side effects while maximizing symptom control.
- Help in exploring and developing psychological coping strategies that may reduce the need for medication.

An alliance is not always easy to achieve. Many people referred to the mental health services are understandably reluctant clients (Figure 13.1) and the negative effects on the working alliance of legal, physical and medical force or coercion cannot be overemphasized. A working alliance represents a mutual commitment and a shared responsibility for the direction and outcome of therapeutic care. This is most likely to be achieved where power

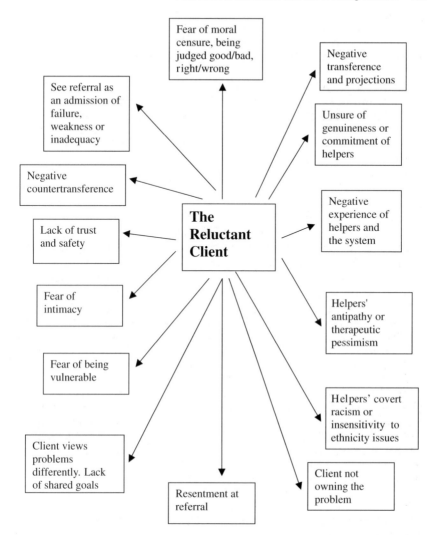

Figure 13.1 Some common factors underlying a reluctance to engage in a working alliance

is recognized as a significant dynamic in the relationship between client and professional helper.

Much Madness is divinest Sense -
To a discerning Eye -
Much sense - the starkest Madness -
'Tis the Majority -
In this, as in All prevail -
Assent- And you are sane -
Demur you're straightway dangerous -
And handled with a Chain -
Emily Dickinson (1830–1886).

Ryan's story *(Theme: non-adherence to care and treatment)*

I've been in and out of hospital eight times since I was seventeen. Once they kept me in about six months. I know that I'm not right if I don't stay on my medication and I know that I'm not right if I do. That's all they seem to worry about, whether you've taken your medication or not. They want me to go to Parkside (a local mental health resource centre). I won't because it's full of older people and nutters. I think hospitals and nurses and doctors make you worse. I pray to the Lord Jesus and I believe in guardian angels. There is a place called Arcadia; it's over the mountains somewhere, perhaps it's in the Himalayas. I've had enough of schizophrenia, I've been in hospital eight times, I've had injections and tablets and it's made me worse. So I don't want to see psychiatrists or CPNs any more. You can't get a girlfriend if you've got a mental illness. The woman who reads the news on Anglia TV used to send messages to me. She didn't say my name but she was thinking it. I wrote to her asking her to meet me in Vagabonds Café. It's like all these mobile phones, the air's full of people's voices. You can hear voices all around you sometimes so I have to put on my personal stereo to drown out the noise of people talking. This nurse, right, she was staring at me and after that I couldn't get an erection and I kept thinking I had abused someone. When I was 10 this bloke made me jerk him off. I've never been violent or abused anyone. I try not to look at people because I know they will put thoughts in my head.... This room is alright but I would like a flat. You can't have a dog here. I wanted to paint the walls blue and green which are my favourite colours but they said I couldn't. I spend a lot of time in the park. I think I could get a gardening job. I wrote to the hospital telling them I didn't need to see the psychiatrist any more and that I would go and see my GP. I've sacked my CPN. He was asking me about how I spent my benefits. He hasn't got a clue what it's like living on benefits.

Harry's story (mental nurse with an assertive outreach team)

I've been working with Ryan for about 6 months now. It has been difficult for the service to engage with him for several years. Every so often he likes to give you 'the sack' and refuses to see you. It's Ryan's way of asserting his power and having some control over his life, which must seem, at times, to be ruled by others. What I'm trying to do is to have a different kind of contact with him, trying to normalize it as much as I can. His life had become so dominated by his illness that it's become difficult to see anything else. I've been trying to relate more to the Ryan that has dreams, interests, strengths and talents. He does get quite thought disordered and hears voices a lot of the time. But he usually manages to retain some coherence despite his thought excursions, and he deals pretty well most of the time with the voices. When they are particularly bad he has in the past come up to the hospital and asked to see a doctor, but now he's afraid of being admitted again and doesn't go there. In total he's spent about three years of the last eight in hospital, the longest was six months. Over that time he's just become more and more exiled from an ordinary life, which is what he desperately wants. He often talks about these utopian mythological places like Arcadia. It's as if he believes he can step out of his world and into a promised land where all is well. It's usually these times that he 'sacks' us and goes into denial about his vulnerability.

Often people who have their first episode of schizophrenia in their late teens lose out on a lot of important development. This is true of Ryan – he's 25 but often he seems more like 17. I see my relationship with him as being more like a mentor than a psychiatric nurse. I'm trying to persuade him to use his local health centre for his fortnightly depot and to see his GP if he needs additional medication to help him through a crisis. What he needs at these times more than anything is someone accessible to talk to and help him deal with any current difficulty. He knows how contact me and has done this when there have been problems. Last time was when he had gone to the police station complaining about people accusing him of abusing children, which hadn't happened. He does sometimes suffer threats and abusive comments from people when he behaves oddly in public places and this can precipitate these paranoid anxieties about being accused of sexual abuse.

I try to respect his wishes when he sacks me and step back, but usually I can arrange to meet him in a local café. We have a mutual interest in dogs and I will take my labrador up to the park and walk him with Ryan. What I'm hoping to do is to persuade Ryan to get involved in one of the nature conservation projects going on in the area and also help him pursue an application for a flat in a supported housing project. It's often these efforts to help in some practical way that leads to a willing engagement with the service, rather than one that is coercive.

Self-enquiry Box

Reflect on a person you are working with, with whom it is difficult to develop an alliance and who presents as a 'reluctant client'. Which of the factors in Figure 13.1 play a part? What else is influential? Now consider how you worked (might have worked) with the client to overcome this barrier.

14 Endings and the working alliance

There will, for every client and mental health professional, be endings to negotiate. The way in which this final phase of the working alliance is managed can be of great psychological significance. As Clarkson (1989) says, 'Every goodbye which is well done in the present can re-evoke and retrospectively help heal incomplete goodbyes in the past.' It is not uncommon for previous experiences of separation and loss to emerge in the end phase. Feelings of rejection and abandonment that have their origins in earlier relationships are transferred on to the present relationship. Strong feelings of anger, fear or sadness may surface. I recall one rather abrupt insensitive ending which resulted in my car being sprayed with engine oil and the sides being badly scored by a hurt and angry client.

With longer-term relationships, a planned, phased withdrawal from a working alliance, keeping the door open and making sure the client knows how to contact the service again, can make the transition easier. This transition from professionally-orientated support to social support can be difficult for many clients. Some will seek to meet their needs for affiliation through continued contact with an ex-patient subculture. This can feel less challenging socially – there is no requirement to account for an important part of their experience and there is less risk of rejection. It can also be of positive benefit to be with people who share your psychiatric experience and to know something of the struggle that may be needed to stay in recovery. But for others, maintaining contact with other users and ex-users is a threat to their self-definition and they prefer, at the risk of painful social isolation, to integrate into the wider community.

It is important to allocate sufficient time to endings. One of the issues that may arise in the end phase of the working alliance for both client and helper is a difficulty in letting go. There may be regression into helplessness, neediness, and uncertainty. Symptoms and problems may reappear. The helper may collude in this process if the relationship meets an unacknowledged need to be needed, so that the client is not allowed to reclaim adult autonomy and independence. It may be that the helper's own deeply held fears about standing alone in the world will be projected on to the client who is then not allowed the dignity of risk. There are echoes here of separation issues in parent–child relationships. The reverse of this can also happen where clients withdraw prematurely to avoid the emotional discomfort of endings. Mental health professionals, too, may end relationships abruptly, 'pushing clients out of the nest before they can fly', on the pretext of avoiding the client's entrapment in a dependent relationship but, at a personal level, as a defence against their own anxieties around dependency issues.

For some people, ending their contact with a professional helper can be experienced as a relief. There is for many people a stigma about being helped that can undermine their self-esteem and sense of their own adequacy. As Barham and Hayward (1995) put it, 'for a person to ask for help, even to admit to himself that help is needed, is to confirm feelings of incompetence and humiliation'.

Andrew's story *(Theme: endings and the working alliance)*
By the time I came out of hospital the second time, my relationship with Justine had finished and I had to find somewhere to live. A social worker helped my get a council flat. He was nice enough, used to call and ask me how I was doing. He was concerned about how I was spending my day. I was spending most of my time in the flat, just going to a local café for my meals, not meeting many people. I got so I didn't bother to tidy the flat or myself very much. I felt demoralized and humiliated really, being on benefits with no prospect of work. In a way him visiting made things worse. I needed to turn over the page on that chapter of my life. Being ill had really shaken my confidence and I needed to prove to myself I could manage. Prove to myself that I was not a mental wreck or a psychiatric case. I got so I rather resented the visits and resented him for being so damn capable and having it all.

There is a need to acknowledge and deal with the feelings and unfinished business that endings evoke, to acknowledge regrets, disappointments, resentments or guilt, as well as any feelings of satisfaction and appreciation. If important feelings are left unexpressed, it can be difficult to let go and move on. This can be as true for helping relationships as it is in personal relationships. During the end phase clients will often look back on their journey through a period of distress and disruption in their lives. There may be a feeling of having 'got somewhere', of improvement in their sense of well-being, in relationships and life skills, in their self-esteem and confidence. Reinforcing what the client has achieved can be a helpful counterbalance to self-doubts that often emerge about their readiness to cope. Allowing time to do this is also important to the helper's sense of competence and worthwhileness.

Therapeutic stocktaking at the end of the working alliance can also be about accepting the 'good enough'. No therapeutic intervention offers a panacea for all life's trials and tribulations. This does not mean that people should abandon cherished dreams and aspirations, however it is worth noting the prayer attributed to St Francis of Assisi:

> God grant me the serenity to accept the things I cannot change
> The courage to change the things I can
> And the wisdom to know the difference.

Self-enquiry Box

In the morning the day is born,
In the afternoon it fades,
Then it disappears all at once.
When this happens
Don't think we took it back,
Don't think that.
The day appears,
Then comes the night.
It will always be this way.
Don't think it will always stay
Dark when the night comes,
That we stole the day from you.
Don't be afraid.
It will always come back.
From Van Over R. (1980) Sunsongs

- *Sit and maintain a quiet focus on the poem.*
- *Brainstorm a list of words associated with endings and beginnings.*
- *Take one word that has some resonance for you.*
- *Put the word into a sentence beginning with 'I'*
- *Put the sentence into a paragraph.*
- *Sit and maintain a quiet focus on the poem.*

Part

3

The therapeutic use of self

Introduction

Part Three of the book goes beyond the working alliance to examine the other characterizing elements of therapeutic relationships identified by Clarkson (1995). What is being proposed in this part is not that mental health professionals should all become therapists, but that we should all be more aware and intentional in how we engage and interact with service users, if we are to be able companions on their recovery journey.

Chapter 15 looks at the psychodynamics of helping relationships and, in particular, explores the phenomenon of transference and counter-transference. Relationships with mental health professionals often provide a blank screen on to which clients project feelings and unresolved issues from other significant relationships in their lives. Similarly, professional helpers bring their own unacknowledged emotional legacy to the relationship, which also becomes part of the unfolding drama. An awareness of what is being acted out in the helping relationship can be important, both in developing and sustaining the relationship and in providing a fulcrum for change.

Chapter 16 explores the reparative, replenishing role of mental health professionals in long-term relationships with service users, a role analogous to parenting. It is argued that through working awarely with this dynamic in the relationship, healing and personality development can take place.

Working in enabling ways with service users involves developing helping relationships in which there is more mutuality and equality than in conventional 'expert-led' relationships. It is a relationship characterized by being real in the relationship rather than role bound. In Chapter 17, the significance of person-to-person interactions as a catalyst for constructive change and some of the ethical dilemmas that working in this way can raise, are examined.

Chapter 18 considers the nature of spiritual care and psycho-spiritual overwhelm as a source of distress. Many people, both public figures and ordinary individuals, relate to others in a way that is infused with spirituality. By this I do not mean to suggest some pious act of caring, more the ability to communicate deeply, in warm, accepting, understanding ways; ways that transcend barriers such as disability, ethnicity, culture, education, class and poverty.

Chapter 19 throws some light on to the shadow side of helping. We would like to think that it is primarily an altruistic motive that draws us into professional caring. Yet it is often our own unmet needs and unresolved issues that prompt us to engage in such work. If we are to work in ways that help people in their recovery, we need to be aware of how our own needs and distress distort our attempts to help others.

15 The dynamics of therapeutic care

Transference is a psychoanalytic concept that describes a key dynamic in helping relationships. It is a phenomenon in which one person, the client, unconsciously experiences the helper as if they were someone else – a significant figure, such as a parent, from their past. What are transferred are the feelings and fantasies that belong to this previous relationship, which may be of a positive or negative nature. There may be feelings of love, affection, pleasure, admiration, concern, desire; or feelings of anger, resentment, bitterness, mistrust, guilt and envy. What distinguishes these feelings from everyday emotional transactions is that they are inappropriate and too intense. As a helper you have a sense of being responded to as if you were someone else (Perry, 1991).

It is important, however, not to interpret every intense emotional transaction as transference. The client's response might be a very understandable reaction to the helper's attitude or behaviour. For example, the client may feel understandably angry when faced with a helper's authoritative, superior attitude, or envious and resentful towards a helper who appears to have all the things in life which the client most desires, but which seem beyond their reach. It is entirely reasonable that a client might feel love and affection and sometimes, sexual desire, for a helper who has supported them in a warm, concerned, understanding way through a challenging period in their life.

The helping relationship provides an ideal screen on which to project these feelings, the caregiver often becoming a significant temporary attachment figure (Byng-Hall, 1995). How these are managed has importance for the helper, whose sense of self can be inflated or deflated by the buffeting of these projections, and for the outcome of the therapeutic alliance which may be undermined. Transference is not, however, a phenomenon that is exclusive to the therapeutic process. It occurs in everyday life between one person and another, between an individual and a group and between an individual and an institution. The script for our ways of relating is laid down in our early formative relationships. Insecure attachments to caregivers during those early years may lead to these insecure attachment patterns being played out in adult relationships.

If transference is not too strong and does not disrupt the relationship and interfere adversely with the helping process, then it may be sufficient simply to acknowledge that some transference is likely to be taking place. Rogers (1986b) takes the view that interpretation of transference is unnecessary and unhelpful. He argues that if the helper is able to demonstrate accurate understanding and acceptance of what the client is experiencing in the here and now, with no interpretation or evaluation, then 'the transference attitudes tend to dissolve and feelings are directed towards their true objects' (p.133). Rogers seems to be suggesting that what we project defensively is what cannot be faced and accepted as part of ourselves. If the helper can contain and accept the projections without getting caught up in them, then they can be taken back and owned by the client who relates them to their true source.

Sometimes, however, in order to deal with a difficult dynamic that has arisen from the client's transference, it may be necessary to engage with the client in a more challenging way – what Egan (1994) describes as immediacy. Immediacy involves focusing on and exploring what is happening here and now in the relationship between helper and client – in the relationship as a whole or in some segment of dialogue. An awareness of a replicative script being played out can be a starting point from which the client can begin to recognize this as a pattern that tends to disrupt their relationships. At a deeper level, a connection may be made with the origin of that behaviour in early experience. The relationship with the helper may, for example, be idealized by the client who surrenders all autonomy and seems to expect the nurse magically to intervene to make life better. Alternatively, the relationship may be one in which the nurse is experienced as detached, pre-occupied and not to be bothered. The client always waits for the nurse to initiate contact and expresses guilt about making demands. In another scenario, a client complains about other mental health workers, seems jealous of other clients and has a need to know about the nurse's personal relationships. All of these scenarios would make it difficult to work effectively with the client in an adult-to-adult way if they remain unaddressed. Failure to recognize and work with transference is thought to be a common reason for unsuccessful treatment (Watkins, 1989).

In transferential relationships there is some risk with people who become distressed and disturbed in a psychotic way. Transference is rather like a personal drama being played out with the helper cast in a role. As in the theatre, the client needs to appreciate the 'as if' quality as the unfolding drama. There is a danger that this may be lost in people who are very psychotic with the helper becoming confused with the object of the transference (Brown and Pedder, 1991).

It is not possible to avoid transference completely, but it can be minimized. This can be achieved by refusing the parent role and engaging with the client in an adult-to-adult way that re-asserts the working alliance. Reality testing is also a way of reducing the distortion of reality that transference induces. Raising the client's awareness of the here and now – 'Is it true that no one listens or cares about you?' helps to achieve this. Dis-identifying from the transference object is also sometimes a necessary intervention – 'You seem in a way to be confusing me with your father. I am not your father and it might be helpful to remind yourself of the ways in which I am different.' This can help to realign the relationship so that a more adult–adult transaction is possible rather than parent–child.

Withdrawal and the inability to engage in social or therapeutic relationships may also be seen as transferential (Clarkson, 1993). It can sometimes be that what the client is transferring is the experience of invasive, neglectful or abusive parenting. Building up trust with such clients can take a long time, but it is through the experience of a caring relationship in the here and now that they learn how to be open to nurturing relationships in everyday life while protecting themselves in more appropriate ways.

Joanna's story *(Theme: transference in the helping relationship)*
Joanna is a 19-year-old unmarried woman with a 5-month-old baby daughter called Rebecca. She has spent the last 2 months in the Mother and Baby Unit at her local mental health unit being treated for puerperal psychosis.

Joanna's early life was characterized by two key losses. First, her parents separated and divorced when she was 10 months old, since when she has only seen her father intermittently. Second, her mother had to work, which meant she and her 2-year-old brother spent much of their early life with a succession of child-minders. Her mother struggled on with very little support and was treated by her general practitioner for depression. When Joanna was 4 her mother began a relationship with another man. Her mother was 'captured' by that relationship and became less accessible to Joanna and her brother.

When Rebecca was born Joanna seemed to project all her own neediness on to the baby providing it with oversolicitous mothering. In the months that followed, Rebecca became increasingly fretful and difficult to satisfy, confronting Joanna with her fear that she was an inadequate mother and, at a deeper level, with the fear that she would never find the love and care she needed for herself. This seemed to precipitate a profoundly hopeless and troubled state of mind in which she developed unusual ideas about the baby and herself. It seemed to Joanna that Rebecca was not her child and she withdrew from her, on one occasion referring to her as the cuckoo. Her belief was that her baby had been given to a childless couple by social services. She showed no distress about this, believing that they would be able to give the baby everything. She became preoccupied with the ideas that she was 'bad inside', that all her 'goodness' and strength had gone into the baby.

During her hospitalization, Joanna has developed a transferential relationship with Hannah her primary nurse who is about the same age as her own mother. She has found it difficult to cope with Hannah's shift patterns and days off, frequently thinking that she must be to blame in some way for her absences and seeking reassurance that she hadn't done anything wrong. She tended to idealize Hannah, seeing her as kind and caring and other staff as hurtful and unpleasant. Often she would try to stay in proximity to Hannah and to other staff when Hannah was not on duty and would often 'collapse' on to staff as if wanting to be held.

The nursing care Joanna received created a scenario on which she projected and played out some of the undealt with issues from her own childhood. Hannah found helpful to give portions of boundaried time, when she could give free attention to Joanna. She was conscious of feeling drained by the demand of being constantly needed. She was able to challenge Joanna's elevated view of her and the contrasting negative view of other staff, helping her to see that this represented how she thought about herself and Rebecca. Slowly Joanna began to re-own and affirm her own 'goodness'. From this more integrated, if fragile position, she was able to accept Rebecca's contentment and demands and reconnect with her maternal feelings.

Countertransference is concerned with the helper's feelings and fantasies about the client. There is no general agreement about the nature of countertransference which, like transference, is part of the social transactions of everyday life. One way of talking about it is to think of it as being proactive – what the helper transfers on to the client from their own past, or reactive – the responses the client induces in the helper.

In its proactive form, the helper relates to the client in a way that is reminiscent of a previous, significant relationship. An example of this is seen in a helper who finds it difficult to be sufficiently assertive in working with clients. In supervision, the helper is able to link this with his need for parental approval, which was conditional on being 'nice' and 'compliant'. Another example is of a helper who, in supervision, acknowledges strong feelings of anxiety and guilt towards a client who has recurrent mental health problems. These were feelings she was able to connect with her own parentified childhood where she had to care for a chronically ill mother.

In reactive countertransference, helpers might find themselves experiencing feelings of anxiety, helplessness, despondency or anger for which there were no identifiable reasons in the helper's life. These feelings may be what the client has difficulty in acknowledging and expressing in himself, which he excludes by putting them out on to the helper – a process called projective identification in psychoanalytic psychotherapy. This ability to resonate with the client's emotional world, communicated in largely unconscious ways, is clearly a useful window on to the client's inner emotional world, if helpers can stay sufficiently aware of what is theirs and what is the client's.

Another example of reactive countertransference can be seen in a helper's tendency to project their own vulnerability or helplessness on to a client, seeing the client as more dependent than they actually are. In this process, the helper is able to distance himself from his own neediness. Meeting a need for power or esteem may also be a hidden motive in the helper's overcaring and overbearing approach to working with clients.

Sometimes as helpers we may over-identify with clients and avoid areas that are similar to our own problems or avoid feelings that are difficult for us to acknowledge and deal with in themselves. The other side of the coin to this is that we work on issues we ourselves need to work on vicariously through the client. So, for example, the client may be asked to carry and work on our own losses as well as their own.

Countertransference is also seen in our reaction to the transference of a client, for example by taking criticism to heart, or being seduced by a client's expressions of love or sexual desire. Perhaps, more commonly, this form of countertransference is seen in the reaction to a client who gives out dependency signals with the helper becoming the protective, nurturing parent. This is, of course, not necessarily an unhelpful complementary role but, if the role is occupied in an unaware, fixed way, it can limit the client's opportunity for personal growth.

We need to guard against any tendency to label every feeling we have for a client, whether positive or negative, as countertransference. Sometimes strong feelings are the authentic here and now responses of one person to another. Rogers (1967) regards 'the full experience of an affectional relationship' as being an important element in the helping relationship for some clients, which may lead to significant learning about the self and others.

This brief section on countertransference underlines the value of both personal development work and supervision as part of the training experience of professional helpers working in the mental health field. It is only through this experience that we can minimize what Heron (1990) calls 'contaminated helping' – that is, helping that is adversely affected by our own agendas. The mental health professions have, until recently, failed to recognize the duality of the personal and the professional in the helping role and have neglected to make provision for this in training and support. It is precisely because personal needs and feelings are denied at a personal and organizational level that we attempt to deal with them vicariously in caring for others. Hawkins and Shoet (1989) makes the challenging observation that effective helping arises out of our willingness to examine our own motives and that in doing so, there is less likelihood of 'the psychiatric client having to carry our own craziness'.

Tony's story *(Theme: countertransference in helping relationships)*
One of the things I noticed quite early in my relationship with Adrian was that he often made reference to similarities between his father and me. I think this made it difficult for him to trust me enough to let me into his life initially. I suspect he must have been wondering whether I would be another critical and ultimately abandoning 'parent'. I was putting in a lot of time with Adrian helping him to open out his life but even so I found myself feeling guilty that I wasn't giving him enough time and leaving him at the end of one of my visits often felt like a small betrayal. I also felt annoyed because I thought he was expecting too much of me and seldom showed me any appreciation. The other thing was I found myself feeling quite anxious about confronting him verbally about his behaviour or encouraging him to take risks in facing situations I knew he would find challenging. We were tending to stay in fairly safe territory.

Taking this to supervision I began to see that some of these feelings had relevance for me and my life. It seemed as if I was accepting his transference, trying to be the 'good father' that he wanted, but could of course never be. I was also picking up his resentments about how his father used to come, stay for a short while, then go, just like me. Not seeing the bigger picture, Adrian's resentment was leaving me feeling both guilty and annoyed.

My uneasiness about challenging Adrian is partly that I am aware of his vulnerability to quite overwhelming paranoid anxiety and I don't want to go too far too fast. But I think this gets overlaid with my own fear of criticism and ridicule that I experienced in my relationship with my father. This causes me to hold back from making interventions.

What I feel now is that we deal with these undercurrents more of the time. If I find myself avoiding, I will look at it with Adrian and explore whether we are colluding. I've tried to dis-identify from Adrian's father by getting Adrian to identify some of the ways I'm different from him. I've also encouraged Adrian to acknowledge the feelings that arise in the 'here and now' of our relationship more of the time and to relocate some of those feelings in the 'there and then' of his past, where that has been appropriate.

Self-enquiry Box

Reflect on the following questions. How might these reactions impose limitations on the process of helping?

- *Do I require affection, approval, appreciation, regard, to be liked, in my relationships with clients?*
- *Do I need to take charge, be authoritative, feel important, be protective, be prescriptive, in my relationships with clients?*
- *Do I find it difficult to allow closeness in my relationships with clients?*
- *Do I see people as individuals or do I have a tendency to label and stereotype people?*
- *Do I feel uncomfortable with certain issues and feelings that arise in my conversations with clients? Are these issues and feelings I need to deal with myself?*
- *Do I catch myself being oversolicitous in my care of people?*
- *Do I feel resentful towards the involvement of carers or other members of the multidisciplinary or multi-agency team in the care of the client?*

16 The therapeutic use of self in developmentally needed or reparative relationships

It has been recognized for many years that one of the helping, healing roles that nurses play in their relationships with clients is that of surrogate parent. As Peplau (1988) puts it, 'permitting the patient to experience older feelings in new situations of helplessness, but with the acceptance and attention that encourages personality development, requires a relationship in which the nurse recognises her surrogate role' (p. 57). Clarkson (1995) sees the developmentally needed relationship as one that 'provides a reparative or replenishing relationship where original parenting was deficient, abusive or overprotective'. The theoretical underpinning for a surrogate role has come mainly from the psychoanalytic stream of ideas on human development and the therapeutic process. In the UK, the ubiquitous influence of the medical model has limited the impact of these ideas on psychiatric nursing practice mainly to therapeutic communities. A notable example is a model of psycho-social nursing that has evolved at the Cassel Hospital (Griffiths and Leach, 1998). Here not only nurse–patient relationships, but the whole social matrix of the community, has developed as a 'culture of enquiry'. The client's difficulties in living are revealed, contained and explored in the daily life of the community and a newly emergent self is nurtured.

Development can be seen as a life-long progressive unfolding of our potential, as human beings and as unique individuals. The emergent self grows and flourishes in a loving, nurturing, encouraging environment, in a way that expresses itself in a sense of well-being. In an unfavourable environment, where the emergent self is not prized and nourished, development will be restricted, weakened and distorted in a way that expresses itself in increased vulnerability and dysfunction.

One of the most significant, research-based theories of human development is attachment theory (Bowlby, 1969, 1973, 1980, 1988). Attachments can be said to lie at the heart of family life. They create bonds that can provide care and security across the life cycle. They can evoke the most intense feelings of joy in the making or of anguish in the breaking and can lead to problems if they become insecure (Byng-Hall, 1995). Attachment behaviour reflects the human need to be close to significant others on whom, in early life, our physical survival depends. For the majority of children, between 57 and 73% (Byng-Hall), attachment to one or more caregivers provides a secure base from which to explore the world with a degree of trust and confidence and for the self and self-esteem to flourish.

For others, those who do not receive 'good enough' parenting, insecure attachment patterns may develop and future relationships be undermined as the result of the replication of these early 'scripts'. The need for attachment and a secure base continues throughout life (Ainsworth, 1991). The knowledge that someone is concerned for you, and has you in mind, supports autonomous, resourceful behaviour, even when an attachment figure is not immediately available. This has significant implications for mental health professionals who, in the context of a caring relationship, often become a temporary attachment figure for their clients. If this dynamic can be worked with in an aware way, then the opportunity exists to do reparative work with the client.

Self-enquiry Box

Gather some small objects together. Objects you have in your pockets or a bag will do. Choose objects to represent yourself and members of your family. Arrange them in the form of a family 'sculpt', that is, a placement pattern that says something about your family system. Try not to deliberate too much at this stage – go with what intuitively feels right.
  You might like to try a family 'sculpt' representing:

- *Your family of origin, when you were a pre-school child.*
- *Your family during your school years.*
- *Your family when you were an adolescent/young adult.*
- *Your family as it is now.*
- *Your family as you would like it to be.*

  Ask yourself:

- *How have the 'sculpts' changed over time?*
- *What have been the important transitional points?*
- *How have I and others in my family, been affected by these transitions?*
- *What do the 'sculpts' have to tell me about my attachment relationships and patterns?*
- *What needs to happen for my family system to change in the way I would like it to?*

Many situations may undermine the capacity of a family to provide a secure base.

Fear of losing or the actual loss of an attachment figure. This may be as the result of the death of a parent or parental separation and divorce. It may be in the form of threats to abandon the child or the use of conditional love to control the child.

The attachment figure is unavailable. Long-term illness in a parent, either physical or psychological, may mean the parent is unavailable or only intermittently available as an attachment figure. In this situation some children will take on a 'parentified' role, becoming caregivers and attachment figures for their parent. While this role reversal may be appropriate later in the life cycle of the family, in childhood and adolescence it can restrict a young person's growth towards independence, making it difficult to separate. In other circumstances a child may feel excluded by another child or the other parent, who has 'captured' the attachment figure.

Scapegoating and misidentification by attachment figures. In some families a child will become the focus of blame for the family's ills and may come to act out that role. In other circumstances, a child becomes identified with someone else in the family, the 'black sheep' or someone with whom the parent has or had a difficult relationship, which is then re-enacted in their relationship with the child.

Abusive relationships with an attachment figure. The most damaging example of a situation that undermines attachment is where a child is emotionally, physically, or sexually abused by someone they would naturally turn to for security. They may feel unable to turn to the other parent for protection for fear of the consequences or because the other parent is unwilling to hear.

Many of these early experiences can be re-enacted in helping relationships, which prompt a replication of 'old scripts'. It is not uncommon for clients to have anxieties about being abandoned or to not feel cared for, despite the attention they receive from their nurse, and of course it can never be enough to make good what was missing from the parenting they received. It is not uncommon for adult survivors of childhood sexual abuse to feel that they have not been heard or believed by professional helpers with whom they share this experience. There is, unfortunately, sometimes a basis in the here and now for this perception. Hearing the client's story can be painful and difficult and the response to it can be muted or incredulous. The client may then begin to feel unheard and unprotected by the nurse just as they were unprotected by significant adults as a child. The currents of powerful feelings – hate, anger, anxiety – that may surface, can create in staff both a strong need to care, but also at times, a sense that they themselves are being abusive.

There is an issue here about the importance of believing clients' stories, even though occasionally they may be fabricated. Early experience may be 'known' at some level and have a profound influence on the behaviour of the client in the here and now, without them necessarily being able to recover the memories of formative experiences or the thoughts and feelings they gave rise to. There can be a number of reasons for this. First, some experiences can be too painful and disturbing to remain in awareness and are shut out of consciousness. Second, parents will often deny or discount a child's experience so that the child is no longer sure what to believe or whether what they are experiencing has validity. Bowlby (1988) gives a number of examples of psychologically distressed adults who, as children, witnessed a parent's suicide but were told that they had died from other, more 'natural', causes. Children may be repeatedly told 'to be grateful', 'to think yourself lucky' or 'you've got nothing to be unhappy about', by parents who find their children's hurt, anger or sadness an uncomfortable echo of their own unacknowledged pain. The consequence of this is that children will begin to disown their discounted thoughts and feelings. Finally, we want to believe that our parents are good parents. We want to believe they love us and are protective towards us. Not to believe so, even when a child's experience is of frequent neglect or rejection, is too threatening.

It can be seen from this brief comment on what is a complex process that there are implications for mental health professionals. It would be easy to deny or discount key events in the client's history if we are not able to stay open and be a validating witness to their unfolding story. If we cannot hear what happened and contain the distress for the client, then it is unlikely they will be able to face that experience. They will not be able to begin the task of re-evaluating it, so that it is no longer such a powerful source of distress, and no longer has such a limiting and disruptive impact on their life.

Attachment theory conceptualizes a process by which we internalize models of our attachment figures and of ourselves in relation to them, which then becomes part of self. What we experience as self is a reflection of the way significant others have behaved towards us. Thus, if we have been cared for in a way that was predominantly loving and sensitively responsive to our needs, we are likely to have internalized an image of ourselves as both a loving and lovable person. If the reverse was true and the care we received was predominantly insensitive, an overly adapted self is likely to develop, which is lacking a sense of self-worth and we will be demanding and insecure in our relationships with others.

While the 'psychological mechanics' of the process differ, there seems little difference in the significance given to attachment figures in the development of the self, between the psychoanalytically orientated views of D.W. Winnicott (see Phillips, 1988) and Alice Miller (Miller, 1990) and ideas of humanistically-orientated writers. Rogers saw the unconditional positive regard of others as being a core condition for the development of what he called the organismic or true self. In other words, if our emergent self is accepted and prized, it is likely to flourish. On the other hand, if we experience rejection, disapproval, or conditional positive regard, the expression of our selfhood is likely to be overlaid by a false self. The false self may enable us to survive and gain some attention and positive regard, but at the cost of a growing alienation from our authentic being. It is not just positive regard from others that we need. We need to feel good about ourselves and if this need is not met it is difficult to function in the world. As Thorne (1992) puts it, 'Our capacity to feel positive about ourselves is dependent on the quality and consistency of the positive regard shown to us by others, and where it is selective (as to some degree it must be for all of us), we are victims of conditions of worth' (p. 31). Positive regard from others is internalized and becomes a sustaining sense of self-worth that enables us to recover from the wounding life experiences of disappointment, failure, rejection and loss that inevitably come along. If our inner core of self-esteem is low, then we are vulnerable to the misfortunes of everyday life and they may overwhelm us with feelings of worthlessness. The alienation from our true self is maintained by our negative self, which continues to censor any expression of the true self that does not meet our internalized conditions of worth. It may, for example, be very difficult for some people to acknowledge certain feelings or needs, because to do so would seem to undermine their sense of self. The negative self can, for many people, be punitive, critical and impossible to live with. They frequently feel a sense of not being good enough in various dimensions of their lives as their organismic self seeks expression.

Self-enquiry Box

You might find it useful to explore aspects your own negative self. One way of doing this is to consider the many shoulds, oughts and musts we all carry around, that can have restricting and limiting effects on our personal growth and undermine our self-esteem.

Write twelve open-ended statements beginning with one or more of the following:

I should...........................
I ought...........................
I must...........................

Now complete the statement with whatever comes to mind. Don't deliberate, go with whatever comes up.

Example

I should know
I ought to be happy
I must do better

Now examine your statements. Ask yourself:

- *Which ones am I most drawn to?*
- *Is this a value that I can own and try to hold to in my life?*
- *Is this a value that I continue to subscribe to but no longer accept as being relevant to my life now?*
- *Where does it come from?*
- *How does it affect the way I feel, think and act?*
- *Do I want to discard it altogether or change it so that it is less prohibitive?*

Bowlby sees development proceeding along a number of possible paths, some leading to adaptive behaviour, others leading to increased vulnerability and maladaptive behaviour. Whether a child is securely or insecurely attached in his or her relationship with significant caregivers is seen as a key factor in determining which pathway an individual takes. Patterns of attachment established during the early years of life tend to persist and will be replicated in other attachment relationships a person makes as they journey through life. While there is some persistence, the developmental pathway is not seen as unchanging, since secure bases provided by other attachment figures in childhood, adolescence and adult life can provide an emotionally corrective experience that enables people to move from an insecure to a secure pathway.

In talking about the therapeutic stance in developmentally needed relationships, Bowlby identifies a number of 'therapeutic tasks'. First and foremost is the need to create a secure base from which the client can begin to explore his or her inner and outer worlds and share thoughts and feelings. The mental health worker will therefore need to be with a client in a way that is accepting, respectful, attentive and reliable and will also need, as far as possible, to see and feel the world through the client's eyes. Important to the experience of a secure base is the ability of the professional helper to contain a client's anxiety and distress. This psychological holding takes place when the mental health professional is experienced as an accessible and supportive presence in the client's life and as someone who communicates a genuine concern and care, who is not critical or rejecting, but stays with the client in their distress, does not react against it by, for example, giving extra medication, but reflects on it and tries to understand it. This is analogous with the way young children are held and comforted when frightened or distressed. When this happens, anxieties begin to subside and the client is less likely to act out their distress in disturbed, problematic ways. Gradually the client learns that intense feelings, fears and fantasies can be contained, reflected on and made sense of, with the expression of disturbing thoughts and feelings in disturbed behaviour being correspondingly reduced.

The secure base may be difficult to achieve and maintain. Insecure attachment patterns express themselves in the therapeutic relationship along with transferential feelings and fantasies. For example, a client may withdraw if he feels the nurse is getting too close for comfort. This happens not because the client wishes to end the relationship, in fact the very opposite. Instead it will be an attempt to maintain the relationship at a distance he or she feels able to bear. Another example might be a client who senses the nurse's emotional reserves are low and that he is unable to provide the emotional

---

Geoff's story *(Theme: reparative relationships)*
Geoff Reeves is a 27 year old who has had frequent contact with the psychiatric services since the age of 18. He has been diagnosed as having a personality disorder and is usually referred in a depressed and suicidal state. His threats of suicide are often of a dramatic and alarming nature, including dousing himself with petrol and threatening to set himself alight, or on another occasion threatening to jump off a motorway road bridge. He drinks heavily and sometimes takes street drugs.

Central to Geoff's early history was, at the age of 8, finding his mother dead, having committed suicide by cutting her wrists. His father, a morose man, who showed little interest in him, began drinking heavily after his wife's death. Geoff was subsequently brought up by an aunt, his mother's sister, who cared for him in a dutiful way but with very little emotional warmth. He left her care at sixteen and lived on the streets in London for a while, where he found some sense of belonging to a 'family' group. The traumatic loss of his mother and the insecure attachments to his father and his aunt left Geoff feeling abandoned, unlovable and 'a jinx'. This latter image of himself, which became embedded in his psyche, originated from his aunt who often told him he was 'jinx on all our lives' and seemed to scapegoat him for things that went wrong in her own family. There was very little family discussion of his mother or her death and he can only talk in a very vague, flat way about his early relationships.

Geoff's relationships with girlfriends have usually ended as a consequence of his demanding and possessive attitude and an excessive need to please the object of his affections. He reacts to any distancing or disapproval in the relationship with prolonged, withdrawn, angry, grief stricken silences. He is currently unemployed and a lack of work is a major preoccupation. It is difficult for Geoff to attribute this to the insecurity of many jobs these days and the ebb and flow of economic circumstances, rather than to his own lack of worth and personal rejection. Crises have often followed the breakdown of a relationship or the loss of a job.

Geoff is currently living in a hostel for young adults with severe emotional problems and attends an outpatient therapy group. The hostel community and the group have provided a secure base for Geoff to begin to recognize and explore the patterns of behaviour that replicate themselves in such a disruptive, distressing way in his current life and relationships. It is difficult at times for both the group and the community to contain his unresponsiveness and his brooding, threatening anger and there is concern when these episodes occur about the risk of self-harm behaviour. Despite these anxieties, the group, the hostel community and Geoff's key worker have been able to maintain a matrix of caring relationships that is allowing Geoff to begin his developmental tasks. There are careful and sensitive limits set in relation to drinking and drug taking, violence and being present, but beyond these conditions of care there is a prevailing sense of unconditional positive regard towards Geoff which is helping him to acknowledge his own worth and value and appreciate himself more. Geoff has surprised himself by discovering a sense of humour. This allows him to laugh at certain frustrations and disappointments, for example, not getting a cleaning job at a local supermarket, a let-down that would previously would have undermined his sense of self and precipitated feelings of hopelessness and desolation.

nourishment needed. Their relational pattern might be to become more demanding in response to anxiety about being 'pushed away'.

Once a secure base has been established, the client may feel safe enough to begin to explore some of the difficulties that arise from their patterns of relating and reacting. I do not see this as 'doing therapy' in the formal sense, although it is a form of 'social therapy': being with the client in different settings, participating with them in the activities of everyday life and using opportunities to engage in purposeful conversation with a client about the issues that create problems of living. Issues arise in the context of living with others, working with others, taking recreation with others and managing the responsibilities of everyday life. The more involved the nurse is in the social matrix of the client's life, the more attuned they can be to the social transactions that take place. These everyday transactions (and sometimes the transactions between the nurse and client) provide 'here and now' examples of old scripts – the past in the present. If these patterns can be recognized, people can be supported in improvising new ways of relating and reacting that are not influenced so strongly by past experience. In the light of the experiential learning that comes out of an ongoing reflection on the 'here and now', old scripts are updated.

In applying attachment theory to the therapeutic process, a particular reference is made to the significance of the client reconnecting with and expressing feelings associated with their experience of attachment relationships (Bowlby, 1988). Often stories of neglect or abuse will be told in a flat, impassive way that gives little hint of how the child in the story felt. Miller (1990) emphasizes how children adapt to parental needs and conditions for love and approval, to such an extent that feelings such as anger, hate, jealousy, anxiety and unhappiness are disowned. This leads to the development of a false self in which our emotional being remains largely unacknowledged and unexpressed. In an empathic, accepting, containing relationship it becomes possible to re-own that lost part of self. Bowlby suggests filling in the 'emotionally blank' story by empathetically engaging with the hurt, angry, sad, frightened child and articulating those feelings. Doing so can

Angela's story *(Theme: reparative relationships)*
I suppose I'd always known it, but never really faced it. I'd been very depressed for about 5 years and had several admissions to hospital. There were other problems as well. I used to get panic attacks and I was very thin, anorexic really. In some ways I didn't mind going into hospital. I always had this feeling that I would be safe there and that this time they would help me. I didn't talk much about my childhood to the doctors or nurses – nobody asked really.

I began talking about it with my CPN. She was a bit older than me, someone I trusted and felt comfortable with. I was telling her about the last time I was in hospital and this male patient came into the female dormitory one night and tried to get into bed with a young girl. I remembered lying there feeling very frightened and not being able to go and get the night nurse. Then I began to talk about how I'd felt like that when I was a child and not being able to tell my mother that my two stepbrothers were sexually abusing me. I couldn't believe it was me saying it, in fact I couldn't believe that what I was saying was true. But Kate (CPN) listened and took what I said seriously. I think she said something like, 'You must have felt very frightened and very alone.' It seemed like she had really heard me and was concerned for me in a way my mother never was. After I'd told her I felt very quite panicky but stifled it, holding it inside, not able to show it. That was the first time. Since then we've talked about it often and it's been very painful emotionally. There were times when I had this fear that she would forget to come and I remember feeling resentful about all the other patients she had to see. I suppose I just had this great need to feel protected at that time. I remember feeling quite angry with her and feeling let down in a way that I can see now I was never able to feel towards my mother. I suppose I'd begun to idealize Kate a bit and it was good for me to recognize that she wasn't perfect, just as parents are not perfect. It helped me to feel a little more forgiving towards my mother and to understand how difficult it was for her. As well as talking, she asked me to write letters, from myself as a ten-year-old girl to myself as an adult and then to reply. It sounded daft but I found it helpful. I was able to express a lot of thoughts and feeling that were quite difficult to talk about. It also helped me to care for myself and to say to my ten-year-old self – 'You were not responsible'.

I've started attending a group for adult survivors who have been abused as children. I'm learning that it wasn't my fault, that I didn't deserve it and that I'm not a bad person. I'm also beginning to learn to trust people and to be a bit more confident and assertive. Looking back I now see my depression as that ten-year-old girl feeling abandoned and frightened, reminding me that she was there and needed to be taken care of.

give clients a powerful sense of being heard and of it being safe to own and discharge these painful feelings.

Bowlby describes the role of the therapeutic helper as being a companion to the client in their exploration. The client is seen as the 'expert' on their own experience who with support and occasional guidance can discover for themselves the true nature of the models that underlie thoughts, feelings and actions and begin the process of restructuring them. Growth and recovery are seen as a naturally occurring process – 'Fortunately the human psyche is like human bones, in its inclination towards self-healing' (Bowlby, 1988). The job of the therapeutic helper is to provide the healing conditions. Similarly, Winnicott was more concerned with care in the service of personal development than cure. He saw the therapeutic process as holding the client's conflicts and distress while development and resolution took place. For Winnicott the significant moments in therapy were when the client 'surprised himself'. Perhaps it is this capacity of clients to 'surprise themselves' that mental health professionals attempt to facilitate through their helping relationships.

Any theory can become dogma and impose itself on an attempt to understand the client's experience. While attachment theory as a basis for practice has arisen from the experience of clinical practice and has been rigorously tested by research studies, like all theories it still does not capture the lived experience of the individual client. As Moore (1996) puts it, 'Each person is a mystery never to be completely understood'. No theory will explain the mystery of being that person. What is much more important is being with people and allowing the mystery that is both our lives to be enacted and better understood.

The person-to-person relationship

This is a relationship between helper and the person seeking help that has the most in common with the social relationships of everyday life. It is a helping relationship in which there is more mutuality and equality. A person-to-person relationship requires us to be 'real' in our interactions, which means being more open and truthful and bringing more of ourselves into the social encounter. It is potentially the most liberating and nurturing of all the helping relationships both for the client and helper, but also one of the most difficult to manage. It requires a significant shift in attitudes – from seeing people as psychiatric patients who are suffering from pathological syndromes and needing treatment to seeing people who are experiencing, and need help with, problems in living. If this is to be more than mere tokenism, then it requires us to relate to people using the mental health services in a different way. It means recognizing that the needs people present with, while they may be more urgent and sometimes desperate, are not qualitatively different from our own. It means facing the possibility that professional helpers do not know best. It means working within more diffuse boundaries than is the norm in therapeutic relationships, replacing a quasi-parental role with a more fraternal one.

The person-to-person relationship is more about being than doing. It is a basic philosophy rather than a technique, which involves being with people in a way that creates a climate for growth and change. Carl Rogers, the originator of person-centred counselling, described this way of being as relating to others in a way that is genuine, accepting and empathic. When it is lived, it connects us with our core selves and frees more of our potential for living. When it is lived in our professional relationships, it facilitates others to engage in self-exploration, self-discovery and constructive change. This remained a central theme in Rogers' writing and research for over 40 years. In a recent review of the research and literature on person-centred therapy, Borzarth (1993) concludes there is little evidence to refute the claim by Rogers that if professional helpers can communicate in an authentic, accepting and empathic way with clients, then this creates the necessary and sufficient conditions for change.

The application of a person-centred approach to helping has been given some prominence in psychiatric nursing literature over the last 30 years (Reynolds and Cormack, 1990). Nurses trained under the English National Boards 1982 syllabus, which identified the core skills of mental health nurses in person-centred terms, had some introduction to the person-centred philosophy. It is unlikely that nurses currently taking modularized diploma and degree courses will have sufficient exposure to the person-centred philosophy for it to become a lived experience. Its values – genuineness, acceptance, empathy – need to be internalized and integrated by the practitioner, so that they become part of him and not a technique or a professional façade. This takes time.

A broad hypothesis of therapeutic human relationships

If I can create a relationship characterized on my part by:

- A genuineness and transparency, in which I am in touch with my real feelings,
- A warm acceptance and prizing of the other as a separate individual,
- A sensitive ability to see the world and himself as he sees them,
  then the other individual in the relationship will:

- Become more integrated and more effective and show fewer characteristics normally termed neurotic or psychotic.
- Have a more realistic view of himself and become more like the person he wishes to be.
- Value himself more highly and become more self-confident.
- Become more understanding and accepting of others.
- Become more open to his experience and deny and repress less.
- Cope more resourcefully and creatively with the stresses and problems of living. (Rogers, 1967 pp 35–37).

Genuineness as a way of being

Genuineness, or congruence, refers to the capacity of the helper to be with the client in an authentic way, not hiding behind any pretence or defence. This degree of 'realness' is hard won. It develops gradually as the result of a commitment to self-awareness, through which the practitioner becomes more in touch with his true self. This parallels the therapeutic process which is also concerned with reclaiming and integrating disowned parts of the self, facilitating the individual's growth towards becoming a fully functioning person. The helper and the client can therefore be seen to be on the same journey. Leitner (1993) argues that practitioners will be unable to take a client further in their personal growth than they have been prepared to go themselves with any degree of acceptance and empathy. There can be no openness to the experience of others unless we are open to our own experience. Congruence is not something that is turned on and off, but is a way of being in the world, a way of relating to others both in our personal and professional lives. It is only possible to live our lives with real integrity when our outer and inner being are in harmony.

Being aware of the feelings, images and thoughts that flow within us when we are working with a client does not mean that we have to disclose everything we experience. In fact, it would not be helpful to do so. What we can helpfully disclose are those feelings, thoughts or images that surface in the here and now as we work with clients and may help them in facing and overcoming the issues that confront them. The key question is, 'What is likely to be the therapeutic benefit of my disclosure to the client'? For example, we may be working with someone who is quite withdrawn and isolated and have a strong sense of hopelessness resonating within us. If this is not our hopelessness, it must belong to the client and can help us connect empathetically with his world.

It can be useful to respond in an authentic way to the client's story and how they present themselves by providing a mirror through which they may reframe troubling life issues or a negative self-concept. This might involve valuing and validating some aspect of the client's behaviour. For example, working with a client who has been sexually abused as a child, it might be helpful to disclose how angry we feel that for that child, that they were not protected and that they should feel to blame. Such openness can allow clients to connect with their own anger and re-evaluate the sense of blame and shame they feel.

Mearns and Thorne (1988) identify a number of reasons why genuineness is important in helping relationships. First, it contributes to the sense of trust a client feels towards the practitioner. Some degree of trust can be gained through role expectation and the knowledge and expertise of the helper, but a deeper sense of trust emerges from a practitioner's honesty and openness. Second, a helper who is willing to be judiciously open about their failings, uncertainties and vulnerabilities, creates a greater sense of equality in the relationship, is more approachable and increases the client's confidence in their ability to understand. Third, the practitioner's congruence models a way of healing that the client is being encouraged to take. A practitioner's acceptance of themselves, their feelings, weaknesses and rough spots, enables clients to own feelings and failings and articulate that experience in a less defensive manner. Finally, genuineness is important because the helper's responses are then an honest reflection of the effect on another person of what the client shares of themselves and their lives. Mearns and Thorne see this as a powerful therapeutic phenomenon that provides the challenge and support which facilitate growth and change.

It is worth keeping in mind that many people referred to the mental health services will have experienced emotional hurt and abuse in significant relationships in the past and may find it difficult to enter into a person-to-person relationship and it may be hard for them to accept the helper's expression of interest and care as genuine. While the person-to-person relationship can be of great benefit, some people need time to work through these issues in a transferential relationship before they can begin to relate in a more person-to-person way.

Being more fully ourselves in helping relationships

It is worth giving some thought to which aspects of yourself you express openly in your relationships with service users you work with. What are some of the issues raised by normalizing relationships in this way?

My feelings of love	*My humour*
My feelings of anxiety	*My spirituality*
My feelings of anger	*My sexuality*
My feelings of joy	*My interests*
My feelings of sadness	*My values*
My feelings of disappointment	*My creativity*
My feelings of regret	*My knowledge*
My warmth	*My vulnerabilities*
My appreciation	*My fallibilities*
My needs	*My lifestyle*
My tactile self	*My personal circumstances*
My playful self	*My caring self*

The ethics of practitioners' self-disclosure

Linked to congruence is the question of what is appropriate self-disclosure for mental health workers in their helping relationships. We first of all need to recognize that reciprocal self-disclosure is a necessary condition for forming and deepening social relationships. It is a social skill without which our relationships would be very superficial and dissatisfying. In professional helping relationships clients are expected to disclose a great deal about themselves and their lives, while helpers disclose very little. When nurses do step out from behind a façade of invulnerability and communicate something of their own experience it is often appreciated by service users. This reciprocity gives the relationship more equality. It is no longer so one-sided, the client gives something back. The fact is that while the dominant discourses in psychiatry created a chasm between those who are diagnosed mentally ill and those who are not, there is in reality no such delineation. What is falsely portrayed as a chasm is, in reality, a small step for any one of us, particularly at those times when our vulnerability is exposed by the challenges and demands of life. The 'us and them' perspective is maintained, partly because we see ourselves reflected in the suffering of others and in our discomfort seek to distance ourselves from what is, however labelled and however extreme, an expression of the human condition. As Sullivan (1953) succinctly put it in referring to people suffering psychosis – 'We are all more alike than different.'

The concept of the wounded healer has recently found some expression in nursing literature (Barker and Davidson, 1998). Nurses have tended to be guarded about their psychological vulnerabilities, often with good reason, as to be open about mental health problems was to risk having doubts cast about their fitness to practise. The generally low use of counselling services located within, or provided by, employing agencies or organizations is an indication that this anxiety remains. The key issue should not be whether mental health professionals suffer emotional problems, some severe enough to be diagnosed as a mental disorder, but what they do with that vulnerability. If it is ignored and denied, then there is the danger of this distress adversely influencing the helping relationship. If it can be faced, understood and healed, then it can be a source of compassionate, empathic helping. Understanding the experience and meaning of a client's distress is likely to be enhanced by an appreciation of the nature of our own wounds and the part these wounds might play in the healing process. The wounded healer has its origins in the shamanistic traditions and beliefs of most ancient cultures. Healers were often people who had suffered, who had visited the spirit world and encountered the spirits responsible for human suffering and returned with the sacred knowledge of healing. There is for me some echo of these ancient traditions in the experience of the mental health professional who is able discover and make judicious use of the healing from his own 'long day's journey into night'.

Acceptance as a way of being

Many people who are referred to the psychiatric services have chronically low self-esteem. This may have arisen out of an early experience of neglect, rejection or abuse. It may have its origins in the experience of conditional love in early life. This may be compounded by social impoverishment and the experience of becoming a mental patient, which reinforces doubts about self-worth and can eclipse an individual's personhood. As Barham and Hayward (1995) show in their study of the lives of people who have suffered a serious mental illness, a person's social identity can become defined by their psychiatric histories.

Whatever the origins of low self-esteem, a person may seek to protect their vulnerable self in defensive behaviour. Given a history of oppressive relationships, it is not surprising that some people may find it difficult to trust the helper and seek to maintain a distance in the relationship or to sabotage the relationship through defensive strategies. They may be withdrawn and guarded with the helper, behave unreliably, question the helper's motives, put the helper down, put themselves down as not being worth helping, behave in aggressive ways, deny or minimize their problems. When clients present in these ways we need to try to stay aware of the hidden agenda – 'Can I really trust this person?' Being with people in an accepting way, if it is consistent, serves the function of helping to create trust and a safe base from which they can begin to explore and make known their inner selves that relate to the world in distressed and disturbed ways. Being with people in an accepting way offers a mirror for them to begin to re-evaluate their worth.

A number of other terms have been used to describe acceptance – a non-judgemental attitude, unconditional positive regard, warmth, respect, valuing, affirming, prizing. It is not an easy attitude to hold to. It can feel difficult to accept some clients – feelings of dislike, disapproval or irritation may be around in the helper's consciousness or just below the level of awareness. This may be based on limited knowledge of the client and if we can focus on understanding the meaning of their behaviour, then any antipathy is usually dispelled and we are able to relate in a more accepting way. Where our feelings persist, it is worth asking ourselves questions such as – 'Who does this person remind me of? Does this attribute that I find so irritating also belong to me? How am I stereotyping this person? How is it that I become impatient/bored/critical/distant when I'm with this client?' Listening openly to ourselves for an answer to these questions can bring into awareness our projections, prejudices and unacknowledged needs and fears.

Mearns and Thorne draw attention to the possibility that the institution within which helping takes place may operate as a conditional culture. The person referred to the psychiatric services, for example, may be expected to be compliant in the helping process, to accept explanations of their problem, gratefully to go along with their care programme and then be discharged. Where people do not conform to this passive role, they may get labelled manipulative, overdependent or resistant. It can be very easy in these circumstances to bend to the pressure of the institutions and become a conditional helper rather than face being seen by colleagues as naïve.

Learning to be with others in an accepting way requires us to be accepting towards ourselves. We must be willing to look at our own needs, vulnerabilities, inadequacies and failings. This can take place in a number of different learning structures that offer a safe and supportive opportunity for self-enquiry. Personal development groups, staff support groups, peer counselling, supervision or personal therapy, are in my view essential elements in the training and professional development of mental health workers. This commitment to self-exploration, self-acceptance and personal growth is not narcissistic or self-indulgent. It springs from the recognition that working in a person-to-person way requires us to show the same respect for ourselves that we wish to show to clients. If we can value and appreciate ourselves, if we can acknowledge our failings and fallibilities, then we can be freer in the way we engage with others.

Empathy as a way of being

Empathic listening is one of the core conditions that contribute to effective alliance. It means being able to enter the landscape of another's world, to see it, as it were, through his or her eyes. It means being sensitive to the flow of feeling we find there, to the meanings that make up this person's perception of the world. It means being able to communicate that understanding accurately.

Empathy is much more than a communication skill, although it is often taught as if it were simply that. It is a process in which we are able to put aside our own frame of reference and experience the other person's world as if it were our own. Empathy is an essential ingredient in human relations. It is the social cement that holds families, communities and societies together. To enjoy good relationships is to be empathic with others. Where individuals or groups have a discordant relationship with others, with their family, with society, then invariably that quality of empathy is missing from their social transactions. We develop this interpersonal quality as we grow up and grow older. The toddler becomes sensitive to the moods of its parents, we identify with our friends in their joyfulness and miseries, we immerse ourselves in another's world in our most intimate relationships and as parents we become attuned to the feelings and needs of our children. The images in art, in film, in literature and music also draw from us an empathic response. At times, however, this human quality remains blocked in our interactions with others. In a professional context, it can feel safer to stay within our own frame of reference than to become involved with the client's meanings and feelings. This leads to helping that comes too much from the head and not enough from the heart – we need both.

How do we become more empathic? A useful place to start is to pay attention to the quality of our listening. Am I listening with my attention free enough to really hear, to hear not just the words, but the meanings and feelings that may lie beneath them? Am I open enough with those with whom I have a working alliance, to communicate what I experience as I hear their story? If I can be more in touch with my own experiences of joy and despair, anxiety and security, attachment and loss, hope and despondency, self-worth and doubt, then, paradoxically, I am likely to be more receptive to this experience in others.

We are all engaged in the same struggle of being human with all the joys and sorrows of the human condition. As Carl Rogers reminds us, the deeper we go the more universal human experience is. This is not to say that my experience of, say, the loss of a parent will be the same as yours. It is important to guard against the tendency to project our own experience on to others and mistake it for empathic insight. But, having experienced the emotional pain of loss, does give me a reference point to help me find you where you are. As Kierkegaard observed, ' If you really want to help somebody, first of all you must find him where he is and start there. This is the secret of caring' (cited in Davis and Fallowfield, 1991). As we enter the client's world and sense some of the confusion, anxiety, anger, helplessness, sadness, etc., we might find there, we must try to stay aware that this feeling is his or hers and not ours. It is all too easy to overidentify and take on the client's feelings.

Rogers considered empathy often to be an intuitive response to the experience of another person. 'There are times when I am listening to people when ideas or images surface as if from nowhere into my consciousness. I find that it is usually worth trusting your intuition enough to share these thoughts with the client.' This can be done in a tentative way: 'The thought occurred to me . . .' or 'I have this picture, I'm not sure whether it will mean anything to you or throw any light on what's going on in your life at the moment.' There seem to me to be different types of knowing. Cognitive knowing – a logical, analytical knowing – is the dominant form in our culture. Other forms of knowing – emotional, imaginative, intuitive knowing, which are a function of the right brain – are undervalued in Western society. Cultivating our intuitive, imaginative potential can, I believe, prove a valuable asset in developing a working alliance with clients.

An important issue to raise here is that while there is a great deal of universality in the way we experience the problems of living, there is a significant element that is culturally determined. It would be arrogant of me to assume I could empathize fully with the experiences of people from ethnic minorities.

Why is empathy so important in skilled helping? First, empathic responses help the flow of conversation. It helps people articulate what is often difficult to put into words. Second, it is very reassuring to be understood and accepted. People often feel isolated with their worries and concerns. There is an awful sense of alienation in the belief that nobody will understand. This leads on to the gathering sense of hopelessness and despair which underlie many acts of self-harm and suicide.

Being understood gives a person a sense of having an ally. From that position they are more likely to examine honestly some of the problematic situations that confront them and work at re-evaluating themselves and aspects of their lives. When someone begins to understand and accept my experience of myself and my life, which may seem to me frightening, weak, foolish, bad, bizarre, and can communicate that understanding and acceptance to me, then I can begin to understand and accept myself. I can begin to claim some of the 'disowned' parts of myself. As Carl Rogers puts it, at its deepest level an empathic response works on the edge of the client's awareness.

Self-enquiry Box

Empathy rating scale

Using an interpersonal process recording of a therapeutic conversation, rate the level of empathy in your responses using the following scale:

Level 0   Response shows no understanding of the content, meaning or feeling in the client's experience

Example: You can't expect to stay well if you don't take your medication. It's a worry to your mother and you'll end up in hospital again.

Level 1   Response shows accurate understanding of some of the content and feeling in the client's disclosures.

Example: It sounds quite a worry for you not knowing whether to mention your illness or not, not knowing how people will react.

Level 2   Response accurately reflects back the content and the intensity of feeling in the client's experience.

Example: So sometimes when you see other people talking together, it seems as if you can hear their voices whispering at you, sneering at you, abusing you. I can understand why you would feel upset and angry.

Level 3   This is advanced empathy that tunes into what's just below the client's level of awareness. The meanings and feelings that are expressed covertly in the clients speech and behaviour.

Example: I'm wondering if all the tension you feel now and that you feel before you harm yourself is something to do with not feeling you can claim attention for yourself. You are never sure whether people care about you or not?

Note the question mark at the end of the examples. Empathic responses may inadequately or inaccurately capture the client's experience. Empathic responses are an attempt to reflect the client's frame of reference – not the helper's. We are saying is this how it is? Although example three could be construed as an interpretation, it comes more from a felt sense of the client's experience rather than from the helper's theoretical reference points.

The person-to-person relationship is in step with the emergent user-centred culture in mental health care. It strikes an opposing stance against the determinism and reductionism of medical model psychiatry and psychoanalytic practice in which the power and expertise reside with professional practitioners. Rogers (1986a), in one of his later papers, emphasizes the importance of trust in person-centred helping. He argues that distrust permeates our institutions including, I would suggest, mental health care. Professional practitioners feel impelled to explain the presenting behaviour in terms of one unproven theoretical perspective or another, to set goals for people and develop strategies and techniques for meeting them. The person-to-person approach has more trust in the resourcefulness of the individual to find his own meanings and way of being. The helping process is concerned with creating the conditions in which people feel able to become more who they are, less constrained by defensive, maladaptive behaviour and able to meet their needs more effectively. This emergent self is revealed in the context of a relationship which is safe and accepting. The helper rejects the role of expert, becoming instead a companion to the client in their search for a way forward. Barker *et al.* (1997) reflect a similar view; psychiatric nursing is seen as concerned with 'establishing the conditions necessary for the person's unique growth and development which involves of necessity the person's adjustment to, or overcoming the life problems associated with, psychiatric disorder' (p. 663).

The person seeking help and their families may of course carry a wish/ hope that the helper will be able to offer some panacea that will make them feel better and will make life better. But often their lives have been full of 'experts' whose expertise has made no appreciable difference. They still suffer chronic or recurrent distress and disturbance which, at times, are overwhelming and disabling. Often their diagnosis, treatment and mental patient status has added to their disabilities. Disillusionment with 'experts' and an awareness of their own budding resourcefulness and responsibility for their own lives, marks the growing edge of change. For some people the continued use of high doses of neuroleptic drugs and a career as a mental patient can seem to smooth out life, make it less of a struggle. But in doing so, mastery over the challenges of everyday life is forfeited and with that a considerable measure of autonomy, self-worth and satisfaction. Helping can ultimately be a hindrance if it does not encourage and respect autonomy.

Mae's story *(Theme: realness, warm regard and empathy in helping relationships)*

Mae is a 47-year-old woman who has been a service user since her mid-twenties, when she was diagnosed as suffering from a manic depressive disorder. It is her lows which are most disabling and distressing and she has made three suicide attempts to end what she describes as the 'numbing misery' of her episodes of depression. Although there is no clear cyclical pattern to Mae's disorder, the worst episodes have tended to occur during the spring. She has always resisted a diagnostic label and has been a reluctant though mostly compliant self-medicator.

Mae recognizes two selves: her 'dull grey self', which seems dominant and recurrent and her 'coloured vibrant self', which emerges briefly and usually as a prelude to a depressive swing. She does not understand why her dull grey self should have such a grip on her life. It seems to Mae that if these two parts of herself could merge, her personality would have more balance.

Mae's personal and family history is that she is the daughter of a white English mother and a black Afro-American father. Her parents never married and she was adopted shortly after her birth. She grew up in a white middle-class family with her two brothers by adoption. She remembers her childhood as unremarkable yet one in which she always felt her parents' love and approval was conditional on her meeting their expectations and standards which, as she grew older, led to frequent arguments and a gradual distancing in their relationship. This was compounded when at 16 she became pregnant and her parents arranged for her to have an abortion. Mae believes that this confirmed for her parents that they had 'taken on a wild child' who 'wasn't the daughter they had in mind'. Mae carries an emotional legacy from that period in her life which hasn't been fully resolved and seems to trouble her increasingly as she moves through her middle years, childless and not in a permanent relationship.

Mae's CPN, Gloria, has been involved with her and her care for the last three years. Their relationship began with the development of a working alliance in which the goals included helping Mae to recognize and manage her depressive thoughts, feelings and behaviour more effectively and to contract with her some strategies for maintaining her safety when suicidal ideas became too intrusive. The relationship now seems to have deepened in a way that seems helpful and respectful to Mae and more involving and satisfying to Gloria. She feels her relationship with Mae is more like a friendship, though both recognize that they are meeting in a professional context and that it is Mae's issues, feelings and needs that are the focus of their interaction. Recently they have talked a lot about what it means to be childless and the emptiness and loss Mae has expressed resonated for Gloria with her own experience of being a surviving twin, an only and lonely child. Drawing on this emotional experience she is able to relate in an empathic way to Mae's story.

Gloria's experience as a black British African-Caribbean woman raised Mae's consciousness of her own Black identity and helped her identify with the richness of black American culture. There seemed to be an important association, for Mae, between this largely unacknowledged part of her identity and the 'coloured vibrant self' that emerged during her 'highs'. Mae talked about a deeply held, but seldom expressed fear, that she had been 'given up' because she was black. She talked about her unknown father in idealized terms and reconnected with painful feelings of hurt and anger towards her birth mother which had been intensified by having to 'give up' her own child.

The warm regard and realness of Gloria's relationship with Mae is helping her to gradually to 'feel at home with herself'.

The ethics of involvement

The person-to-person relationship requires involvement. This raises some interesting and important questions. How can I have an authentic relationship with someone that I am paid to engage with and perhaps would not choose to spend time with socially if the context were different? How is it possible to draw boundaries between this type of relationship and a friendship? What constitutes overinvolvement? What if clients become attached to me? What if I become attracted to the client sexually and what if they become attracted to me? How can I end a person-to-person relationship?

Perhaps the key to all these questions is honesty and openness. Yes, I am paid to engage with the person in my care, but that does not mean that my interest and care has to be any less genuine. Yes, it is a role but it is a role that is infused with myself to the extent that it becomes the role of no role. I want to be with a person in need in a real or authentic way that earns their trust. If I reveal so little of myself in my helping relationships that people do not experience me as a person, there is little on which to build a trusting relationship. To engage in a way that is emotionally distant seems to me to dehumanize the relationship and care then becomes a mechanical act.

I want to relate to people in a fully human way and that means bringing along my feelings. It means that I will like and feel a great deal of affection for some people and, at the other end of the continuum, will at times feel antipathy towards others. It means that I will often be deeply affected by the painful struggles and adversities that people face. It means that I will at times feel angry at the behaviour people exhibit or at the social injustice and oppression that they experience. It means that I will at times feel anxious when faced with the distress and disturbance the client brings and experience a sense of powerlessness when faced with the complexity of a client's problem. It means that at times I will feel sexually attracted to the clients with whom I work.

It does not mean that we have to express or act on the feelings that surface in our consciousness. There are good reasons why we should not. First, clients do not want the burden of our feelings or the responsibility for our needs. They need to feel that we will be able to contain their distress and that the problems and needs they bring are paramount. Second, people who seek help from the psychiatric services are often very vulnerable, both emotionally and socially, to insensitivity and exploitation. There is a power imbalance in helping relationships that creates opportunities for unethical practitioners to exploit people using the service, materially, emotionally and sexually. The UKCC (1998) in their guide to working with vulnerable clients are very clear:

> 'As a registered nurse, midwife or health visitor, you are personally accountable for your practice and, in the exercise of your professional accountability, must avoid any abuse of your privileged relationship with patients and clients and of the privileged access allowed to their person, property, residence or workplace' (UKCC Code of professional Conduct, Clause 9).

The guidelines go on to raise practitioners' awareness that sexual relationships between practitioners and clients will almost certainly be a breach of the code of professional conduct and subject to disciplinary action and may constitute a legal offence under the Mental Health Act. It cautions practitioners against using their power and influence with clients to meet their own needs or to benefit financially or materially. It questions 'whether it is ever appropriate to have anything other than a purely professional relationship with the client' (p. 18).

These are sensible rules governing the conduct of professional relationships, which are by nature intimate. Boundaries must be set for the protection of both clients and practitioners and as the UKCC (1999) underline in the guidelines on the prevention of the above, this is clearly the responsibility of the practitioner. But, in a caring culture that aims to normalize and 'de-professionalize' helping, the line between what is justified therapeutically and what is ethically questionable is thinly drawn. Is all affectionate physical contact taboo? Is socializing with a client outside working hours always unacceptable? Is a client's attachment to a helper necessarily undesirable? Should a client's sexual attraction to a key worker or a practitioner's sexual attraction to a client be seen as impropriety? Is friendship never permissible? Many clients appreciate a practitioner's willingness to engage in a relationship that has the qualities of friendship (Figure 17.1). What is valued is the ordinariness of these relationships which are anchored in reality and normality by ordinary companionship but in which the client is not exhausted by the helper's desire to help. As Ram Dass puts it, 'The more you think of yourself as a therapist, the more

---

Self-enquiry Box

You may find it helpful to reflect on your current relationships with clients from the perspective of Figure 17.1.
- *Do you find yourself crossing boundaries in a way that allows the qualities of friendship to enter your helping relationships?*
- *Do you experience this as generally helpful or generally problematic in helping people in their recovery?*

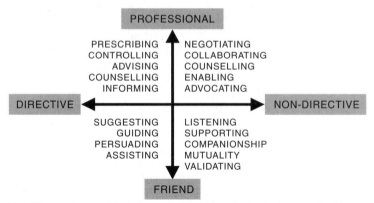

Figure 17.1 Dimensions of helping relationships (adapted from Jackson and Stevenson, 1998)

pressure there is on someone to be a patient'. (Ram Dass and Gorman, 1989). In my view it is possible and often desirable in long-term contact, to bring the qualities of friendship to the helping relationship without losing our discipline and integrity. What turns a committed helping relationship into an 'overinvolved' and potentially unethical relationship, is the intrusion of the helper's needs and feelings, in a way that skews the relationship towards dealing more with those needs and feelings than the clients.

Sexuality in the context of helping relationships can be particularly difficult if it is not dealt with openly. If it is ignored or denied at an individual or team level, and not acknowledged as a commonly occurring dynamic in helping relationships, it increases the risk of practitioners being exposed to compromising situations and to clients being sexually exploited and their trust betrayed. If a client's sexual attraction to a practitioner is treated in a censorious way, they can feel humiliated and guilty. If the practitioner reacts by becoming more distant, the client can feel rejected. These issues need to be brought to supervision and other appropriate staff forums and discussed openly and respectfully, acknowledging the anxiety and uncertainty they can create. This is unlikely to happen if there is gender stereotyping in which male staff are exposed to accusations of predatory sexual behaviour with little recognition that female clients sometimes use their sexuality to seduce and entrap staff. Female staff, too, may be given little support in dealing with the sexual attentions of a client, the implication being that they are to blame for getting overinvolved with clients and leading them on. Gallop (1998) observes that overinvolvement may sometimes reflect both the practitioner's and the client's unmet need to feel 'special', which creates a dynamic for symbiotic relationships that are potentially exploitative. Female staff may harbour rescuing fantasies believing that they, through their special relationship with the client, can save them from destructive behaviour patterns. Clients may respond to this attention by feeding the nurse's fantasy that they alone have made a difference. Relationships in which this dynamic is active, run a great risk of transgressing professional boundaries as the client's emotional demands on the nurse increase. Occasionally male staff may use power coercively to exploit clients sexually, sometimes seeing this as a legitimate development of their therapeutic work. Others may use power in a more paternalistic but none the less damaging way that fosters an emotional attachment leading to a sexual involvement.

Sexuality is part of normal human interaction. Attraction and playful flirtation is an enjoyable element in many social transactions. For some clients, the owning and expression of their sexuality is part of the recovery process and it would be surprising if professional carers were not at times a focus for that sexual interest, given the intimate and caring nature of the relationship. But social signals can easily be misinterpreted, particularly where a client is socially isolated or has pressing unmet need to feel special and for a loving, sexually-consummated relationship. In such a scenario the warmth of a helper's interest and care may be taken as a cue that they are willing to enter into such a relationship. Unfortunately, this so often ends with advances being rejected and the hurt and angry client making formal complaints of sexual harassment or abuse against the nurse. There is a need for us as helpers to be more aware and proactive in reasserting our boundaries and to work through the resulting issues and feelings in an open and supportive way with the client before this degree of emotional investment and sexual interest takes hold.

There can, as we have seen in the previous chapter, be a transferential element to feelings of love and attraction to a professional helper, who becomes the nurturing, protective parent or attentive lover, with whom the client seeks to satisfy unmet attachment needs. However, it would be unhelpful to interpret all transactions between staff and clients in which an emotional and sexual attachment develops as the past in the present. In

---

Rebecca's story *(Theme: over involvement in practitioner–client relationships)*
Rebecca is a recently qualified staff nurse working in an acute admission assessment unit. She is a primary nurse for a group of six clients. She has found herself thinking more and more about Liam, a 27-year-old man with a history of depression and alcoholism, who is in her client group. She has had a lot of therapeutic contact with Liam over the past few weeks and enjoys his mildly flirtatious, humorous conversation and his appreciation of her as a nurse. They have met a few times in the hospital cafeteria for a coffee after Rebecca's shift has ended and she has occasionally been shopping for him, things she would not normally agree to do. Gradually their conversations have become more reciprocal with Rebecca sharing personal information and talking about a recently ended relationship. A friend and colleague, recognizing Rebecca's overinvolvement, mentioned it to her, only to be met with resentful annoyance at her intrusion and Rebecca's insistence that she was quite capable of managing her relationships with clients. The matter was not reported to a senior member of the team and neither did Rebecca bring the issue up in supervision.

She felt that Liam was benefiting therapeutically from their relationship and that she could help him transcend his depressive personality and destructive drinking. During one of their conversations Liam asks her if it would be all right for him to contact her socially when he was discharged. He tells her that he feels considerably stronger emotionally as a consequence of her help, but worries how he will cope when he leaves the unit and no longer has her support.

Following his discharge they meet socially and soon begin dating. After three months they move into a flat together. It is not long before Liam is drinking again and their relationship is in crisis. There are frequent angry exchanges in which he accuses Rebecca of never being off duty, of analysing him and trying to run his life for him. Rebecca decides the relationship is over after he accuses her of seeing other men and attempts to rape her. Three weeks later Liam is readmitted following an overdose taken after several weeks of heavy drinking. Rebecca has no alternative but to report her relationship with Liam to her clinical team leader who arranges for Rebecca to be transferred to another unit. She is required to attend a disciplinary interview at which she agrees to seek counselling and to make the management of boundaries a focus of her supervision.

ongoing caring relationships, in which there is often a social as well as a therapeutic dimension, Eros is bound to enter the interplay sometimes. Where this attraction is reciprocal, it can be very difficult for a practitioner to ensure professional boundaries are not transgressed and it is perhaps too much to expect them to continue working with the client.

18 The spiritual dimension of therapeutic care

The meaning of spirituality and the nature of spiritual care in the context of mental health nursing are probably two of the most important yet largely ignored care themes to emerge as we move into the 21st century. Nolan and Crawford (1997) argue that, in the quest for professional respectability and a scientific knowledge base, we have become disconnected from mental health care's deepest roots: responding to a human being's spirituality. The spiritual dimension of the helping relationship is difficult to define, even if its importance is recognized. One way of doing so would be to describe it as that element in human relationships which transcends people and situations. It is perhaps most apparent in relationships which are empty of the helper's ego and when the client is wholly and fully accepted without any expectations of them to be different.

Nursing claims to have a holistic view of patient care, yet training and practice rarely go beyond the physical and psycho-social to include the spiritual (Dyson *et al.*, 1997). There is a hesitancy and discomfort about engaging people in a consideration of their spiritual needs. This is not surprising as there is a widespread assumption that spirituality and religion are the same thing and that spirituality is therefore the responsibility of the chaplain or leaders of the patient's faith community. Instead we need to recognize that organized religion provides just one (albeit important) way of connecting with and expressing spirituality.

If we are going to work in this holistic way and include the spiritual, we must recognize our own need and take steps along the path of our own spiritual development. In post-modern Britain there is a growing recognition that all kinds of dogmatism are flawed. Science, whether physical, biological, or behavioural, does not offer absolute truths about the meaning and experience of being human and, in a largely secular society, neither does organized religion. Yet the need for one's life to have purpose and meaning remains as strong as ever. Finding answers to the question of what invests our lives with those qualities is part of the quest for a more spiritual life. Often that need surfaces and becomes more compelling at times of crisis. For others a spiritual journey is prompted by a nagging sense of dissatisfaction and incompleteness.

What is spiritual care? In a review of the literature, Dyson *et al.* identify a strong relational theme in spirituality. How I relate to myself; how I relate to others; how I relate to God; and the interconnectedness of these three elements. The first of these, how I relate to myself, is concerned with the question of loving myself. Can I have regard for myself, care for myself? Can I recognize my essential goodness, despite all my flaws and failings? This theme occurs often in the stories of people in distress who seek help from the psychiatric services. It seems that it is as much through the experience of receiving compassionate care, as through psychological interventions, that people come to love themselves a little more. When this happens, it may open the door to an awareness of a universal spirit both within us and around us, which challenges the idea of God as a personified deity, a Supreme Being, occupying some divine realm.

If we reflect a little on the second of Dyson's observations about the relational nature of spirituality – how I relate to others – there can be no doubt that some people, both high profile figures and many ordinary individuals, relate to others in their work and everyday lives in a way that is infused with spirituality. They engage with people in a way that transcends the potential barriers of mental illness, disability, culture, ethnicity, class, education, poverty and communicate understanding, warm acceptance and compassion. There is a similarity here to the unconditional positive regard that Carl Rogers describes as one of three core conditions for facilitating growth and change. Although Rogers spoke out against institutional religion, towards the end of his life he made reference to a spiritual dimension in helping relationships. He describes moments in his therapeutic work when . . . 'my own inner spirit has reached out and touched the inner spirit of others. Our relationship transcends itself and becomes part of something larger' (Rogers, 1986b). In his account of Rogers' life and work, Thorne (1992) refers to a spiritual awakening that for some people seems to occur in person-centred therapy. He concludes that in the process of self-actualization we may discover at our deepest centre the human spirit which is open and transcendent, a discovery which launches us on a spiritual journey and changes our way of being in the world.

The experience of severe mental illness can cut a person loose from their moorings. They feel adrift in unfamiliar seas, in search of landmarks, alienated from others. It can seem, at times, as if the person is lost in chaotic seas of madness. To care well for someone suffering from mental illness is in some way to share their experience, to enter their chaotic world as if it were our own, but without losing the capacity to return to our own moorings. Relating empathically which, Rogers contends, is one of the most powerful elements in the healing process because it brings even the most frightened, (disturbed and chaotic) client back into the human race. If a person can be understood, he or she belongs' (Rogers, 1986b). Respecting an individual's personhood is a moral imperative that must underlie the practice of psychiatric nursing. We have to try to hold on to the person who is trying to make sense of a psychotic experience, whose sense of self and the world have become skewed in confusing and alarming ways. We have to help them communicate what has hitherto been unintelligible, to validate their experience and to treat them as a person of worth. Similarly, Breggin (1996), in writing about the psycho-spiritual care of deeply disturbed persons, emphasizes the importance of the principles of love and liberty in the caring relationship. He argues that healing is facilitated through loving relationships characterized by a 'treasuring of others that is reverent, caring and empathic' and by nurturing and respecting self-determination. Inglesby (1998) suggests that the use of a spiritual/religious lens can help make sense of madness. Religious imagery can be seen as a metaphor that bridges the chasm between ordinary experience and the unintelligible world of the person whose experience is termed psychotic. She argues that mental anguish can be seen as part of a journey of redemption and renewal. For many people, the experience of becoming deeply depressed or lost in the chaos of a psychotic experience can be like a descent into a personal hell. Yet it is a place from which renewal is possible. The hope is in the energy and movement that is locked into anguish and turmoil. As Nietzsche said, 'Only out of chaos may there be born a dancing star' (cited in Inglesby). The hope is also in the willingness of carers to witness and validate the experience of suffering and to provide companionship to people on their journey in search of the truth that heals. It is difficult to return alone and alienation leads to despair and annihilation of the self. The return to a way of being in the world that is different from before is a recovery pathway. What is recovered is a stronger sense of identity and a more authentic and ethical way of being. This is in contrast to a rehabilitation pathway which aims to return people as near as possible to the point from which their descent into turmoil begun. As Inglesby puts it 'the descent may have been necessary to find a path out into the light.'

The third theme to be considered is our relationship with 'God'. As mentioned earlier, a much broader and less restrictive definition of God has been emerging. While many people will seek God and express their spirituality through one of the religious faiths, others begin their journey to their spiritual centre and seek spiritual nourishment through the practice of meditation, through the images of art, music and poetry, through a reverence of nature or through psychotherapy. Perhaps what we are in touch with when we are in communion with God is an essential life force – a force that is present in nature, which may be captured in music and art or found in sacred places and be present in ourselves and others.

The person struggling with psychological disabilities is often dispirited and demoralized. We intuitively know, though this is seldom acknowledged in the professionalized arena of mental health care, that the recovery of the spirit is necessary to the recovery of well-being. The power of the arts and nature to restore the spirit and aid the recovery process has been recognized for centuries. The enlightened care provided for the mentally ill at The Retreat, York, in the late 1700s included what is now sometimes referred to as horticultural therapy, art, music and drama therapy. Yet in modern times this important source of psycho-spiritual healing is available to the few rather than the many. There have been several imaginative schemes to bring the arts into places of healing (see Helping to Heal) which are so often soulless buildings. The use of poems in public settings is an example of the way in which spiritual nourishment can be brought into everyday lives.

There is often an unnamed absence in people's life that cannot be made good by a materialistic, hedonistic lifestyle. Erich Fromm (1993), in his analysis of Western culture in the 20th century, describes a society dominated by the acquisitive motive: we must have success, status, money, qualifications, a bigger house, a better car, material possessions, a husband/wife, children, sources of entertainment. These have become the benchmarks of our worth, from which our sense of self-esteem and the esteem of others are largely derived, with the result that we look for fulfilment from what we have. They may give us some transitory pleasure but they do little nourish the spirit and maintain our sense of well-being. Fromm argues that there is a moral imperative for turning from this 'having mode' and embracing a lifestyle that places more value on what he refers to as the 'being mode', which is concerned with finding ways of being at peace with oneself, with others, and with the world. It is about caring compassionately for others, for the world and for ourselves. When we are being truly human, we are able to recognize the divine in others and in the world and have a greater awareness of the interconnectedness of all things.

In recent years, there has been a growing emphasis on understanding mental health problems in the context of a multi-ethnic society (Fernando, 1995), yet little attention has been paid to the importance of religion and faith communities in clients' lives. In many large urban areas, faith communities – be they Muslim, Sikh, Hindu, Buddhist, or the many denominations of the Christian Church – provide a stronger sense of community and personal identity than any other neighbourhood groups (Copsey, 1997). Religious and spiritual beliefs are profoundly important to many people with mental health problems (Mental Health Foundation, 1997). They provide a source of support and comfort and add a powerful sense of meaning to people's lives. Copsey argues that there is a need for mental health professionals to engage in a dialogue with local faith communities in multi-faith areas in an open way without expecting them to take a Western world view of mental health problems which largely excludes the spiritual dimension of people's lives. Rationalistic, secular beliefs about health and well-being may be difficult to reconcile with the teaching of world religions that put living an ethical life as central theme in the avoidance of suffering. There is a need for mental health professionals to develop a greater sensitivity to the beliefs and practices of clients. The problems of living that people present with, the confused and painful experience they are troubled by, must be seen in the context of cultural and religious beliefs.

If care in the community is to mean more than professionalized care, faith communities that are central to the lives of many service users' lives must be encouraged to become involved in providing help and support and to develop a more informed understanding of mental health problems. For while religion and membership of a faith community is a nourishing experience for most people, for some it can be damaging. Religious doctrine and the attitude of some faith communities have at times left people feeling a sense of blame and failure for having psychiatric problems. Others have felt rejected by their faith communities at a time when inclusion, warmth and support were most needed.

Self-enquiry Box

There are a number of guided visualizations and meditation exercises that are that are helpful in developing a spiritual awareness. You might like to try the following:

Exercise 1. Sit comfortably on a straight-backed chair with your feet flat on the floor. Give a little more of your body weight to the chair. Allow it to support you. Take a few deep breaths down into your abdomen. Allow yourself to settle, to become quiet and still.

Now imagine yourself walking along a path through some fields. The path is gently rising and ahead of you is a hill. The sun is shining and there is a light refreshing breeze. Be aware as you walk of the bird song. Be aware of the flowers among the meadow grass and the breeze stirring the leaves of nearby trees. Imagine yourself crossing a footbridge over a busy stream and following the footpath up through some deep cool woods. You emerge from the woods and follow the path winding round the hill towards the summit. As you walk you stop from time to time to enjoy the changing vista of the countryside stretched out below and to bathe in the peace and solitude of the place. As you approach the summit you become aware that you are about to meet someone, your inner guide – a wise person, connected with the evolution of your life. A person whose eyes express a great deal of love and care for you. Allow yourself to visualize this person. Allow a clear image to form. Now imagine yourself talking with your wise person. Ask about any issue, problem, choice, opportunity, that you currently have in your life. Be open to the answers to your questions, allow them to surface in your consciousness. At the end of your conversation your wise person gives you a gift of symbolic significance to you. Something you need at this moment in your life. Receive what you are given. Thank your inner guide. Now imagine yourself walking back down the winding path carrying with you the answers to your questions and the gift. Picture yourself walking down through the wood and crossing the stream. Walk back across the meadows to the start of your walk.

When you are ready, bring your attention back to the here and now. Consider what you have learned and how you can incorporate this learning into your life.

Self-enquiry Box

Exercise 2. Sit quietly for a minute or so.

- *Become aware of the experience of your body. Become aware of your thoughts without getting caught up in them. Notice your feelings, however faint, without being drawn into them. Now allow yourself to scan your life in the present and the past. Allow your recollections to settle where they will. As you do this, be aware of the effect on your body, your thoughts, your emotions. Experience whatever is there. Now give your attention to developing an attitude of lovingkindness towards yourself. If it helps, repeat to yourself 'May I be peaceful and happy'. Try to maintain this compassionate focus towards yourself for a minute or two. If you find your attention wandering, gently bring it back to an expression of care for yourself.*
- *Concentrate your attention on a friend. Bring them to mind. Be aware of your feelings. Now give attention to developing an attitude of loving kindness towards your friend. Try to maintain this compassionate focus for a minute or two.*
- *Concentrate your attention on a person whom you dislike or who dislikes you. Bring them to mind. Be aware of your feelings. Now give attention to developing an attitude of lovingkindness towards this person. Try to maintain this compassionate focus for a minute or two.*

- Concentrate your attention on a group of people, a community, or a nation, particularly those who are experiencing oppression and adversity. Bring a representative image to mind. Be aware of your feelings. Now give attention to developing an attitude of lovingkindness towards them. Try to maintain this compassionate focus for a minute or two.
- Concentrate attention on the earth, on its sustaining beauty and its abuse. Bring a representative image to mind. Be aware of your feelings. Now give attention to developing an attitude of loving care towards the earth. Try to maintain this compassionate focus for a minute or two.

NB, Initially you may find it difficult to locate your feelings or they may be very faint. Reconnecting with feelings comes with practice. It comes from sitting quietly and becoming mindful of your bodily sensations and from there to the emergent feeling. Giving your attention to a feeling allows it to surface more fully into consciousness. Sometimes you may be surprised by negative feelings. These should be acknowledged without becoming drawn into them. They can be helpful moments of learning about yourself and your relationships and lead to changes in how you relate. It may be difficult to access your feelings of lovingkindness. Recollecting a moment in time when you felt that way or experienced lovingkindness from others may be a way into that feeling state. Above all this exercise requires

19 The shadow side of helping relationships

We would like to think that what draws us into the mental health professions is the motivation to be of service to others, to respond in a skilled and selfless way to the needs of people coming to the service for help. This saintly viewpoint is rightly questioned by Skynner (1989), who suggests that it is often our own unmet needs and unresolved issues that prompt us to engage in such work. He puts forward the view that institutional care, whether it be in a hospital or in the community, can be seen as a theatre in which the helper's needs and issues are played out and satisfaction sought. At best there is some degree of mutuality, with the client as well as the helper getting some of their needs met through the relationship. Skynner is not suggesting that the mental health professions should have in place some ultrasensitive selection process that screens out all but those with the highest motives – who would be left to do the work! What is important is that professionals become sufficiently self-aware as to acknowledge some of their own issues and needs that may intrude unhelpfully into their work with clients. Acknowledged needs can find expression and satisfaction in our personal relationships, unacknowledged needs become demands which may unconsciously intrude into our working relationships. This view is shared by Brandon (1976) who argues that helping others is for some a way of concealing 'desperate personal needs'. We may give care and advice to people which we are unable to give ourselves. We may prop up our own sense of adequacy against the inadequacy of others.

John Heron also takes up this theme strongly in arguing for what he calls 'emotional competence' in helpers (Heron, 1990). By this he means that our own anxieties and distress, accumulated from past experience, should not drive and distort out attempts to help others. He describes three levels of competence:

Level 1: At this level a person's helping is always contaminated by hidden agendas and has an oppressive, hindering, intrusive or impersonal quality of which the practitioner is unaware.

Level 2: At this second level the helper acts in emotionally clean ways most of the time but sometimes slips over into compulsive, distorted helping without realizing it.

Level 3: At this third level the helper slips much less often and more importantly recognizes when it happens and can take steps to correct it.

People who work at this level will usually have done some psychological work on past distresses which gives them more awareness and the ability to act intentionally more of the time.

The second level is widespread among both professional and lay helpers and often leads to 'contaminated helping'. Specific examples of 'contaminated interventions' are legion and can be outlined in relation to the six categories of helping interventions originated by Heron.

Contaminated interventions in helping relationships

Prescriptive interventions

Giving advice when it is not needed; 'taking over', overriding the client's autonomy and responsibility; being coercive and imposing in giving advice; giving moralistic prescriptions – 'you should'; being controlling; not allowing clients the dignity of risk and the right to fail; not allowing clients to say what they need or choose; not being assertive in giving advice and prescriptive care when it is needed; giving advice the helper needs to hear themselves; use of threats or force.

Informative interventions

Not giving information about diagnosis, drugs, resources or legal rights which is wanted and needed; imposing 'mystifying' explanations and interpretations; labelling and stigmatizing clients; not listening to or respecting the client's frame of reference; giving false information; making unrealizable promises of help or promising overly optimistic outcomes.

Catalytic interventions

Asking too many questions; using blocking tactics to control the agenda; attention not free for the client; staying in safe territory, avoiding difficult issues; manipulating the client into being over-disclosing; engaging in a compulsive search for 'answers'; focusing on the helper's issues in the client's story or avoiding them; maintaining a distant professional stance, not fostering any sense of mutuality or equality; sexual or emotional exploitation of a client's transference.

Cathartic interventions

Not reaching out to clients in distress; not 'giving permission' to be upset; discounting or placating distress; talking over a client's distress; missing or ignoring cues to distress just below the surface; pushing people into catharsis inappropriately or too soon; giving 'conditional care'; being overwhelmed by the client's catharsis that finds an echo in the helper's own unacknowledged distress; being controlling rather than containing when clients become distressed.

Challenging interventions

Avoiding or talking around issues because of the helper's anxiety about raising it directly; not raising issues because of the helper's fear of retalia-

---

tion, of hurting the client, or of spoiling the relationship; being apologetic and defensive in raising issues; not being assertive in raising issues so that challenges can easily be dismissed or ignored; challenging clients aggressively or judgementally; swinging from evasiveness to 'hard truths' and back again to evasiveness because of the helper's anxieties; the helper 'overtalks', denying the client the space to assimilate and question what has been said; avoids or anxiously raising agendas that would be difficult for the helper only to find the client accepts them without undue concern; abusive verbal assaults on clients.

Supportive interventions

Support is given in a patronising or insincere way; support is given intrusively, rescuing the client, showering them with help and care when they are struggling resourcefully with their problems; not recognizing and reaching out supportively when help is asked for overtly or covertly; not allowing the expression of dependency needs; holding clients in a dependent relationship, blocking the clients in their efforts to support themselves or draw on other sources of support.

(Source: Heron, 1990)

Self-enquiry Box

- *You may find it helpful to reflect on these examples of 'contaminated interventions' in relation to your own practice. Challenge yourself! We can all recognize ourselves in some of the interventions outlined. Your attention may also be drawn to patterns in your way of relating to clients of which you are not so aware.*
- *Ask your clients what they have found helpful and not so helpful about the way you have worked with them.*
- *You may find it valuable to explore the outcomes of your self-enquiry in supervision.*

Egan (1994) takes a broader view of the shadow side of helping suggesting that alongside the helper's shadow side is the client's shadow side and the shadow side of the helping process, all of which can contaminate and hinder the helping process.

Not everyone wants to be helped or can be helped. The client may seem to engage in a relationship and the helping process with serious intent but does nothing to tackle his problems or seize opportunities offered. This passivity or reluctance has to be acknowledged and explored before there can be any change. Sometimes this centres round dependency needs. A client may have a need 'to be held', to feel cared for to a greater degree and for a longer period than the helper or the multidisciplinary team realizes. They need time to feel that the relationship will provide them with a safe base from which to begin to assert their autonomy and become more effective in meeting the demands and challenges of everyday life. The helper may strongly value independence and self-reliance in their own life and may have personal anxieties around dependency, all of which can have an unnoticed influence on their attitude towards the client. This may express itself in feelings of impatience and blame towards the client for their lack of progress, to which the client may react by retreating further into passivity and dependency.

Clients sometimes manipulate helpers in order to meet their hidden agendas. They may seek to gain the helper's concern by threats of self-harm or actual harm, they may stop taking medication, or not turn up for an appointment, or leave the ward without telling anyone – behaviours which have a powerful impact on professional helpers. Clients may sometimes retreat into symptom behaviour and helplessness and, by clinging to a sick role, avoid the discontinuation of care. Clients may emotionally, and sometimes sexually, seduce helpers in order to meet a need to feel special, to feel loved, appreciated and valued. Clients may be non-engaging and non-compliant with helpers or the service as an expression of their resentment at the way they have been treated by mental health and social services in the past. All these issues can be considered part of the client's shadow side that can hinder the development of helping relationships.

The process of helping also has its shadow side. The history of psychiatry is chequered with examples of abuse. The stigmatizing, disempowering, disenfranchising attitudes and practices of the institutional era of psychiatry still exist in community-orientated services of today. Many long-term users of the services have little choice or say in their care plan and are subjected to under-stimulating programmes of day care that do little to meet their needs for socially valued work and leisure activity. Many users feel hindered rather than helped by excessive doses of neuroleptic medication which often add to their disabilities. In reviewing the evidence for drug-induced disability, Breggin estimates that between 10 and 20% of people treated with the phenothiazine group of drugs will develop tardive dyskinesia.

The professionalization of caring and what Brandon (1997) calls the 'therapeutic egos' of many helpers creates a culture of disparagement where people whose behaviour is distressed and disturbed enough to become the objects of 'expert' attention are pathologized and treated. Personhood becomes submerged beneath the mantle of mental patient and the individual excluded to the margins of society from where it is very difficult to reclaim citizenship. The tendency to pathologize behaviour that deviates from the arbitrary social norm seems to be increasing. The current Diagnostic Statistical Manual of Mental Disorder IV contains 390 categories of mental illness compared with DSM 111 that had 205. It is argued (Coleman, 1998) that rather than representing the advancement of scientific knowledge it reflects psychiatry's encroachment into normal human responses. Life can be a struggle. Happiness is not a divine right. There are no easy answers to the adversities and the pain of living. Yet our culture seems to promote a utopian view that there is a solution to all the problems of being human. This is often reflected in the unrealistic expectations of professional help, held by both clients and helpers, who look for the 'big fix', instead of a small but definite change that results in a problem being managed better rather than resolved.

Like many mental health professionals, I have been slow to recognize my own feelings and needs that have at times intruded in a way that has hindered clients in their journey of recovery. I have at times not been proactive in getting the help and supervision I needed. This is in part the result of my cultural conditioning, reinforced by a work culture that places a high value on independence, self-reliance, stoicism and selflessness. As James Hillman observes, 'We have been brought up to deny our needs. To need is to be dependent and weak; needing implies submission to another' (cited in Hawkins and Shoet, 1989).

Ruth's story *(Theme: contaminated helping)*

Harry is a man of 37 who has suffered from a manic depressive disorder and alcoholism for some years. His key worker, Ruth, visits him weekly providing a supportive alliance within which early relapse signs can be monitored and coping strategies implemented. There is some evidence that Harry is drinking again and he has not been at home on two occasions when his key worker had called. Ruth is aware of feeling quite angry towards Harry for what she sees as his 'deceptive' and 'irresponsible' behaviour. She feels let down by him after all the 'hard work' she's put in. On her next visit she aggressively confronts Harry and threatens to discharge him if he is unwilling to follow the agreed care plan. She leaves feeling unhappy, guilty and compromised professionally.

In supervision Ruth is able to discuss this incident with a senior colleague. She recognizes that an 'over-investment' in problem resolution in her work with clients, is a pattern that often leads to her blaming herself or blaming clients for a lack of therapeutic endeavour. She traces this to her own experience of a much-loved alcoholic father, who both her mother and herself were never able to 'help enough'.

Martin's story *(Theme: contaminated helping)*

Martin is a mental health worker at a supported housing project. He has been Jeannie's support worker since she moved to the project two months ago, after a lengthy period in hospital. Jeannie had been admitted in a disturbed, distressed state of mind, complaining of hallucinations and delusions. She has made a good recovery but is a vulnerable young woman with a pressing need for a secure supportive relationship. She is in her twenties, single and grew up in foster care and various children's homes, following parental desertion. Jeannie tends to search Martin out on the slightest pretext and has clearly become attached to him. Martin feels flattered by her regard for him and plays along with the flirtation that has crept into their conversations, at one level seeing it as a normal expression of sexuality and entirely appropriate in a caring culture that seeks to normalize professional helping relationships. Gradually social excursions become opportunities for discrete intimate exchanges and Martin finds himself increasingly attracted to her. It is not long before Jeannie tells Martin that she is in love with him and clearly signals her willingness to enter into a sexual relationship.

Martin feels confused. He is currently unattached, as is Jeannie. There is mutual attraction that in other circumstances would lead to an emotional and sexual relationship. Yet he is aware of having crossed a professional boundary in allowing a mutual attraction and emotional involvement to develop as it has. He is aware that in the past he has knowingly drawn clients both male and female into enmeshed relationships with his personable attention, only to withdraw defensively when demands began to be made which ethically he could not fulfil. In supervision he is able to acknowledge the feeling of power he experiences when people idealize him and need him in the way Jeannie does now. His supervisor recognizes that Martin's unmet narcissistic needs are intruding in a potentially damaging way into his work with clients.

Self-enquiry Box

You might find it helpful to think about how the two scenarios above might be resolved:

- *In a way that minimizes the distress to the client and enables them to retain some trust in the professional integrity of the service.*
- *In a way that enables the mental health professional to get the support and help they need.*

Part

4

Personal management

Introduction

A recurring theme throughout this book has been the importance of practitioners being committed to their own growth and development. There is a need to avoid the potentially damaging split that so often occurs in professional caring, in which the helper's vulnerabilities, needs and problems of living are denied and only the client's vulnerabilities and neediness are seen.

We cannot be effective as helpers if we live an unexamined life. Knowing ourselves allows us to relate more sensitively and empathically to others, for as Carl Rogers argued, what is most personal is also most universal. To be more intentional and authentic in the way we relate to people is to be less influenced by the unconscious motivations of our own unacknowledged needs and unresolved distress. This final section of the book sets out three ways in which personal management as a vital, integral part of professional development can enhance practice.

Chapter 20 considers the place of personal development within professional education. The first step in this process is developing self-awareness. It is argued that if we remain blind to our own defensive communication patterns, our oppressive attitudes and prejudices, our own needs and feelings, our personal wounds and undealt with distress, then it unlikely that we will be able to engage with service users in ways that will be experienced as helpful and healing.

The energy and resourcefulness we are able to bring to the helping relationship will depend greatly on our ability to take care of ourselves. The high rates of sickness, absenteeism and burnout among mental health professionals suggest we are not very good at doing this. Chapter 21 explores ways in which work related stress can be creatively managed.

Chapter 22 examines the importance of regular, planned opportunities for guided reflection on practice. There are times when our work as mental health practitioners seems hardly worthwhile; when it seems to achieve little; when clients seem lost in their distress. There are times when the experience and problems of living people bring, seem crushing and insurmountable. There are times when we feel impotent, inadequate and drained, with little left to give. It is because helping relationships can be so challenging and depleting, that good supervision plays such a vital part in replenishing helpers and in developing and sustaining competent, creative practice.

20 Personal development in professional education

Relationship skills are the key attribute that mental health professionals bring to their work. Such skills are not easy to acquire and training programmes at pre- and post-registration level need to find creative ways of helping students and practitioners of nursing to develop depth as well as breadth in their skills repertoire. This depth, I would argue, comes from personal development work and should be seen as a prerequisite for effective psychological helping.

Mental health nursing is a process of 'social healing' that seeks to respond to the problems and needs of people, often very vulnerable and troubled people, in a way that helps them move towards a more effective way of being. At its best it is an empowering, enabling process that is rooted in a belief in the potential of people to recover themselves and their lives from enduring and disabling distress. I use the term 'social healing' not with the intention of seeking to relabel caring to give it the status of a therapy but because, to my mind, it accurately describes a core function of mental health nurses. To fill out this role, nurses need a thorough psycho-social training that goes beyond communication skills, beyond psychological strategies and techniques and brings the self more fully into the role. This chapter looks at how personal education, concerned with the 'art of being', can coexist in the academic context alongside a curriculum concerned with 'knowledgeable doing'.

A great deal of professional education is characterized by what Knowles (1991) defines as didactic, pedagogic teaching and learning and is principally concerned with cognitive knowing. Clearly this is not an appropriate way to meet the need for personal development. An experiential, student-centred approach offers a more fruitful teaching and learning style. By experiential learning I mean the active and interactive involvement of people in structures that engage them holistically. The educational process needs to engage people at a feeling, intuitive and sensory level, as well as the cognitive, if they are to become skilled in the intentional and therapeutic use of self. Experiential structures are designed to create opportunities for gaining self-knowledge, for learning how to relate to others in a more authentic way. They are concerned with knowing how to be present with people in ways that are enabling and healing. Learning takes place within collaborative relationships with teachers and fellow students, in which responsibility for the learning process is shared. The underlying philosophy is that of student-centred teaching (Rogers and Freiberg, 1994).

Student-centred, adult-orientated approach to teaching helpfully parallels the collaborative relationship between nurse and client and mirrors the person-centred philosophy of care programmes. Relationships of empowerment need to permeate the culture of caring organizations and the supporting educational culture, involving students and teachers, practitioners, clinical team leaders and service managers, if service users are going to experience the help they receive as enabling and empowering. Power differences need to be acknowledged as a dynamic in all human relationships and managed awarely in a way that are anti-oppressive. In a supportive and empowering educational culture students can take responsibility for determining their learning needs and become resourceful in getting those needs met.

Much of the experiential learning methodology has come from the field of humanistic psychology and from the arts. When used imaginatively and facilitated well, these structures can contribute in an exciting, relevant and effective way to professional development. There is a rich seam of structures to draw on, some examples of which you will have already experienced in this book:

- Co-counselling techniques
- Guided visualization
- Expressive writing
- Journal keeping
- Encounter style personal development groups
- Intrapersonal and interpersonal awareness exercises
- Expressive art
- Role play
- Improvisation
- Mask work
- Storymaking
- Sculpting
- Psychodrama
- Movement exercises
- Meditation.

My own experience of facilitating drama-based experiential groups suggests that personal development that has significance for professional practice can take place in an educational context. An approach to experiential design drawn from drama therapy seems to offer a challenging but safe structure in which students are less likely to become overexposed to the point of vulnerability and shut down protectively. Students find the self-discovery talk and openness to feeling in a cohesive group to be a strengthening and enlivening experience. Such groups can create a context in which inner empathy can develop so that the help offered to clients is less likely to be contaminated by mental health workers' own needs and feelings. Another interesting outcome from this type of educational work is the increase in awareness of the non-verbal channel of communication. The process of helping normally depends heavily on words and we become blinkered to the subtle yet significant messages conveyed by body language. Drama exercises that focus on bodily communication can re-awaken us to the dance of life. Finally, students often observe that they are able to relate in more spontaneous ways as a consequence of participation in drama-based experiential groups. Gersie (1991) suggests that many of us have internalized critical judgements about our capacity to be creative that have blocked our imagination and creative energy. Finding the freedom to be creative in such a group can increase the vitality and spontaneity available for everyday life and relationships.

Key learning experiences reported by students in a drama-based experiential learning group

Giving and receiving support
Increase in knowledge of self
Increased awareness of group processes
Increase in openness/self-disclosure
Affective learning/more in touch with feelings
Increased interpersonal awareness
Increased spontaneity and confidence
Raised awareness of bodily communication
Strengthened ability to process experience reflectively

(Source: Watkins, 1995)

Self-awareness

As Burnard (1990) suggests, self-awareness is the first stage of learning how to use ourselves as therapeutic agents. If we remain blind to our defensive communication patterns, our oppressive attitudes and prejudices, our own needs and feelings, our emotional wounds and undealt with distress, then it is unlikely that our engagement with people using the service will be experienced as helpful and healing. This unknown side of ourselves – the shadow side – will appear like an uninvited guest in our interactions with clients. It is difficult to stop ourselves reacting in a hurt angry way to rejection or criticism from a client if we are blind to our need to feel 'special' in our relationships with our clients. It can be difficult to accept non-compliance if our need for control, and the anxieties that surface if control is lost, has not been examined. It can be difficult to see past the vulnerabilities and neediness of clients if we do not recognize our own needs and fallibilities. It is unlikely that we will be effective in nurturing the self-esteem of others if we have a fragile sense of our own self-worth. We cannot expect to work helpfully with people of a different gender, sexual orientation or ethnicity to our own, if we have not considered the biases that we have inherited from our culture and how they influence our interactions. We cannot create a helping dialogue if we are not aware of the inner distractions that prevent us from having our attention free for people. These kinds of statements about the art of helping seem to me to represent the case for self-awareness and personal development work to be an essential core running through the initial training and continuing professional development of all mental health staff.

Heron (1990) argues that it is important that helpers free themselves from past hurts and develop emotional competence if needs and feelings that have their origins in past relationships are not to spill over into our helping relationships. By emotional competence he means that we will be in touch with our feelings and can both appropriately control and discharge our distress. It means that we have choice; we are in charge of our feelings rather than them being in charge of us. Traditionally, the helping professions, particularly nursing, have sustained a culture which overvalued the control of feelings. To acknowledge feeling upset or, worse, to show that upset, could have resulted in practitioners being thought inadequate and unsuitable. Stress-related problems and burnout follow in the wake of a failure to recognize the emotional labour of nursing and create a culture in which practitioners' feelings are respected (Smith, 1992). We cannot care empathically for people, recognize and respond to their feelings, if we are not in touch with our own. It can be difficult to allow and respond appropriately to a person's distress if we cannot face and deal with our own emotional pain. We may not see the signs of distress in others or, if we do, we may fail to reach out. Alternatively, we may smother others' distress in comforting words and actions, when the safe discharge of distress and the gathering of insight into the context for the distressed reaction would be a more therapeutic response.

Self-esteem

Many people suffer from low self-esteem. Their experiences of life, particularly early developmental and educational experiences, have not allowed them to internalize sufficient self-regard to weather the winds of fortune that blow through life. Their self-esteem is either too externally regulated or internally sensitized. In the former, self-esteem may be frequently punctured by minor experiences of disappointment, let-down and failure that are part of everyday human experience. In the latter, self-esteem is sensitized to particular events, so that an individual crumples when exposed, for example, to criticism or to not being centre stage. Self-esteem is not derived from seeing only our positive qualities and talents and defensively ignoring our flaws and failings. It involves being able to acknowledge our imperfections, changing what we can change and accepting what we cannot. Self-esteem comes from living a life that contains and expresses what we value for ourselves. Sometimes when we feel bad about ourselves it is because we perceive ourselves as falling short of certain standards or values which, if we took the trouble to examine, we would not wish to continue to own. They are values that we have picked up from our parents or teachers or they may have been imposed by our culture.

For the mental health practitioner, a low self-esteem may make it difficult to find the confidence to engage with some clients and sustain a relationship. Doubts and uncertainties will frequently surface about being good enough to do the work. Things that clients may do or say will be experienced as hurtful. Relating to people in an honest way becomes difficult. Some practitioners may feel they have nothing worthwhile to say or feel that they will not be listened to. Others may find it difficult to be open to the appreciation and regard of others.

Personal development work in the context of professional education should sustain and enhance the self-esteem of practitioners. It should develop relationships and educational structures within which a person can become known and feel valued and validated. It should create a forum in which the conscious incompetence of a practitioner can be disclosed as a starting place for development. Clearly, if insufficient trust exists then practitioners are more likely to adopt defensively a position of unconscious incompetence and practise in unaware ways which are potentially harmful. Educational groups that have personal development as a desired outcome, support groups and supervision, offer the opportunities to work on and strengthen self-esteem. An important step in building and sustaining self-esteem is being able to obtain feedback from others.

Self-enquiry Box

You may find it useful to reflect on Johari's window (Figure 20.1) as a structure for developing self-awareness. Each panel of the window represents a way in which our self expresses itself in our everyday lives. Panel 1 is the part of ourselves that we know best and that is known to others – our persona, the self that we commonly present to the world. Panel 2 is that part of ourselves that is seen by others but which we deny or are unaware of. Panel 3 is the part of ourselves that we know of, a familiar companion, but one that we keep hidden from others. Panel 4 is that part of ourselves which is largely unconscious but which expresses itself in our actions and reactions. Generally speaking the wider the open area (1) the more integrated and fully functioning we are.

You might find it helpful to consider:

- how you might become more aware of how people experience you (2). Be open to feedback. Notice any tendency to negate positive feedback or react defensively to criticism. Ask for specific feedback from colleagues, clients or friends whose openness and honesty you trust.
- which aspects of yourself you keep hidden from others (3)? It might be helpful to take a look at the self enquiry box on page 163. What might be the positive outcomes of being more self-disclosing?
- finding out about the 'unknown', largely unconscious, aspects of yourself (4) may involve personal therapy, engaging in personal development in educational groups, developing inner empathy, guided self reflection.

Since drawing and painting are effective non-verbal ways of exploring the Self, you might like to try taking a large sheet of paper, select some colours and draw or paint an image to represent the Self that you present to the world most of the time. Try to allow yourself to paint/draw in a spontaneous way. Don't think too much about it, just do it and see what emerges. There are no prizes for artistic achievement! Take about 10 minutes to do this and then put it aside, out of sight. Take a second sheet and draw or paint an image to represent yourself at times in your life when you have felt most fully alive. You may find it helps to spend a few minutes quietly scanning back on some of those moments in your life. Now select some colours and begin to draw/paint again, allowing yourself to be as free as possible about this. Again take about 10 minutes. Now compare the two. One way to do this is to brainstorm a list of adjectives that come to mind when you look at each drawing. You might like to consider what prevents you being in touch with the self expressed in the second picture more of the time.

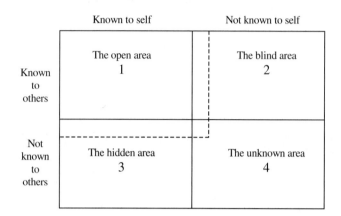

Figure 20.1 Johari's window

21 Taking care of ourselves

Taking care of others, particularly people with severe psychological disabilities, can be demanding and stressful. The energy and resourcefulness that we have to bring to that helping relationship will depend greatly on our ability to take care of ourselves. Professional helpers are generally not good at this, not good at identifying and meeting their own needs. The high rates of sickness, absenteeism and attrition are an indicator of the presence of stress and burnout among mental health nurses (Thomas, 1997). There are several reasons why nurses are not very good at self-care. Often the culture of caring occupations carries an unspoken belief that, come what may, staff cope, so that to acknowledge being stressed or upset is to risk being thought neurotic or unsuitable. The wider culture, too, imposes expectations in the form of gender-linked values and beliefs, such as 'women are expected to put others' needs before their own', or 'men are expected to be tough-minded and strong'. Onyett (1998) observes how 'macho cultures' develop in community mental health teams and contribute to staff stress. There is what he describes as an 'addiction to accomplishment', in which nurses take on more and more work and boundaries around hours worked begin to slip. In this kind of work environment, interaction with colleagues becomes exclusively work-orientated with little time for the kind of informal social contact which can be experienced as depressurizing. At a deeper, more personal level, we are sometimes drawn into helping or caring occupations as a covert way of meeting our own neglected and denied needs. In other words, we give to others what we ourselves need. We recognize in others the vulnerable part of ourselves which is difficult for us to own, and that becomes the hook for projecting our own vulnerability and neediness. Taking care of ourselves starts with owning that vulnerability and neediness and recognizing it as part of the condition of being human.

The challenge in our work can be stimulating. People often say they work better under pressure and it certainly seems to be the case that up to a certain point stress does improve performance. Beyond that point, however, our performance begins to deteriorate. If we are subjected to sustained stress, either at work or in our personal life, and do not adequately de-stress, then we run the risk not only of becoming inefficient and ineffective in our work but also of burnout and ill health (Figure 21.1). We can become so accustomed to living on the down slope, that we become unaware that we

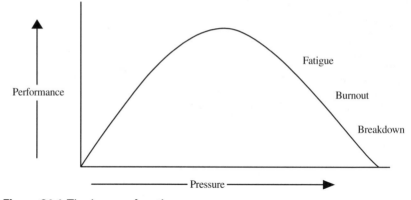

Figure 21.1 The human function curve

are stressed until stress symptoms become so intrusive that we can no longer ignore them.

Hawkins and Shoet (1989) suggest that burnout is a process which begins quite early in the careers of helpers. It arises principally out of an over-attachment or an overinvestment in helping clients. Most of us struggle with the issue of non-attachment. We often lurch between the poles of impotence and omnipotence, feeling a sense of inadequacy and failure at one moment and infallibility the next. Non-attachment does not mean not caring, it means 'I care but I don't mind'. I care for clients compassionately in their struggles to manage the problems of living more effectively. But, if they are motivated to escape from that struggle into symptom behaviour, or for a time seek refuge in a more dependent ways of being, or seek relief in street drugs or self-harm behaviour, then I don't mind. If I did I would soon become disillusioned, demoralized and exhausted. Nurses suffering from burnout show less empathy towards clients, adopt a depersonalizing, cynical approach to care, and minimize contact, seeking refuge in administrative and routine tasks (Santa Maria, 1998).

> ## Self-enquiry Box
>
> *This exercise will help you become aware of how stress affects you. Reflect back on a recent stressful period in your life. Focus on the way in which you were affected. You may find it helpful to categorize your list of personal reactions under the following four headings: physical, emotional, mental, behavioural. Stress tends to have a diverse effect on human functioning. If you find it difficult to identify effects in a particular category, you may be ignoring important signs of stress in your life. Now compare your list with Table 21.1.*

Table 21.1 Examples of the effects of stress

Physical	Mental	Emotional	Behavioural
Headache	Forgetfulness	Discontent	Resisting change/ inflexibility
Indigestion	Poor concentration	Anxiety/worry	Cynicism
Tense, tight muscles, back ache, neck-ache	Difficulties with decision making and thinking things through	Apprehensive a lot of the time	Absenteeism
Sleeplessness		Tearful	Talking a lot
Menstrual problems	Putting oneself down	Hopelessness Irritable, annoyed	Overworking
Diarrhoea	Beating oneself up	Angry more of the time	Losing interest easily Apathy, inertia
Tiredness, exhaustion		Easily exasperated	Withdrawn
Restlessness	Imagining the worst	More despondent, sad, depre	Destructiveness Drinking a lot
Cold hands and feet	Changing one's mind		Insensitive, impatient with others
Trembling	Confused, muddled	Helplessness	Avoiding people
Jumpiness	Dreaming a lot	Resentment	Taking less care with appearance, diet, hygiene
Frequency		High, excitable	
Sweating		Doubt/Uncertainty	
Palpitations			Making mistakes
Tight breathing			Reduced commitment to work
Pallor			Complaining a lot
			Taking work home 'Busy' syndrome
			'Indispensable' syndrome

Stress, like beauty, is in the eye of the beholder. What we find difficult and stressful in our work, others may find less so. It is not so much that situations are stressful but how we perceive them. Take for example a person who, despite having disabling problems, resents the interventions of mental health staff, seeing them as intrusive and unwanted. Try as the staff may, all they get is abuse. Some helpers might find this behaviour very upsetting and stressful to deal with, perhaps seeing it as a personal rejection or a reflection on their adequacy as a nurse. Others may react differently, perhaps seeing the resistance and abuse in a less personalized way, interpreting it as the expression of the anger the client feels about his loss of control over his life or the oppressive care he has received in the past.

Looking after at-risk clients can be very anxiety provoking for some staff. It may be they are the sort of people who tend to anticipate 'the worst' – to catastrophize and, as a result, adopt a very controlling, directive approach to care. Others may be able to take a more balanced view and allow clients the dignity of risk in order to encourage self-responsibility and wise action. Here again we can see how stress can arise primarily from within.

Sometimes the stress we experience has more to do with some previous, perhaps distant, distressing experience, which is in some way mirrored by the current situation. In this case, we might find that feelings of anxiety, anger or sadness can be restimulated by the current event. If we find ourselves unreasonably upset by a particular person or situation, it is useful to ask ourselves, 'Who does he/she remind me of? When have I been in situations like this before?' A client's abusive experience or loss may remind us of our own and if the issues and feelings around that experience have been incompletely dealt with, then we may find ourselves perturbed by the client's story.

Self-enquiry Box

This exercise will help you identify key stressors in your work situation. Look at this list of stressors and decide which apply to you. Add other stressors not on your list that apply in your own work experience.

- *Having no say in what happens.*
- *Frequency of organizational change.*
- *Having to deal with difficult behaviour, e.g. hostile behaviour, self-harm behaviour, non-compliant behaviour, high levels of neediness and dependence, high levels of distress.*
- *Lack of appreciation.*
- *Cynicism and negative attitudes in others.*
- *Lack of progress or slow pace of therapeutic change.*
- *Increasing bureaucracy involved in delivering care.*
- *High turnover of disturbed distressed clients in inpatient settings.*
- *Heavy caseload of clients with complex problems.*
- *Job responsibility unclear or unreasonable.*
- *Being criticized.*
- *Not having appropriate skills.*
- *Getting overattached to residents/residents getting overattached to you.*
- *Lack of support systems within the service.*
- *Having to account for one's work in a multi-disciplinary, multi-agency context.*
- *'Macho' management ethos.*
- *Lack of resources to provide quality care.*

Now rate the items on your list with a high/average/low stress rating. Be aware of the number of high to average ratings present in your current work situation.

Now ask yourself: What needs to change? The situation? The way I think about it? The way I react to it physically/emotionally? Perhaps all three?

Now ask yourself: How am I going to do it? What resources do I have now that I could use? What new strategies could I adopt/learn that would be useful to me?

You may find it helpful to read to the end of this section and then return to this task.

Most of us have a selection of strategies ranging from the ordinary to the exotic, which we use to manage the stress in our lives. I use the term 'manage' as opposed to 'cope with' or 'resolve', because the former implies treading water and the latter is often unrealistic – not all stress situations are resolvable. But what we can do is to manage the stressful situation and/ or ourselves more effectively so that we are mostly on the up slope, making stress work for us rather than against us.

Managing stress more effectively involves answering three questions: What is the problem? What do I want to do about it? How am I going to do it? We have so far been considering the first of these three questions. The second question involves considering what needs to change for me to feel under less stress and pressure. I might decide that what needs to happen is to be able to stay more relaxed in busy, pressured situations or to leave work behind me when I am off duty or that in among the demands of home and work I need some time and space for myself. Perhaps I need to increase the level of support available to me or to reward and nurture myself a bit more, to say what I think and feel about what frustrates me. We can think of these as desired outcomes which, if they were in place, would make a significant difference to our stress levels. Imagining how a situation might realistically change helps us to 'climb out' from under the stress in our lives – to take charge of our lives.

The third question, 'How am I going to do it?' translates these ideas into action. Let's take 'Being able to stay more relaxed in busy pressured situations' as our desired outcome. We might decide that one helpful piece of action would be to join a yoga class to cultivate a more centred approach to life. We could also learn breathing techniques, which could be used at times when we felt under pressure. We might also try building three five-minute relaxation periods into our working day, clearing the mind and letting the tension leave your body even for these short periods helps prevent over-stimulation. At home we could try an Alexander Technique lie down, which is a valuable way of releasing tension and restoring energy. (It involves lying on the floor with two or three paperback books under your head, having your knees bent and feet flat on the floor.) Another strategy we may decide to adopt is to ask for more support from others or to speak to our seniors about an unreasonable workload. These last two strategies may require cultivating some assertiveness skills.

We need to keep in mind when considering how we might take better care of ourselves how often intentions remains just that – intentions. It is helpful to ask ourselves, 'What is going to be my first move? When am I going to do it?' Enlist the support of someone to help reinforce your commitment. Be aware of some of the things that might prevent you from getting started and from keeping it going. Ask yourself, 'How could I reduce these obstacles?'

Self-enquiry Box

This exercise will help you become more aware of your support system.

Take a large sheet of paper. Represent yourself in the centre. Map out all the people and groups that you experience as supportive. Put important sources of support close to you and less important ones further away. Draw in arrows to show whether support is one-way or mutual.

You may find in doing this exercise that you have a good, sustaining support system in your life right now. Conversely, you may find it is some-what limited. Ask yourself, 'Do I give out a lot but don't receive? Am I open

> to support? Is the support that I get helpful, i.e. not rescuing, imposing or manipulative?'
>   Now ask yourself, 'What are some of the things I could do to strengthen my support system?'
>   'What else, apart from the people in your life, do you draw on for support'?

Remind yourself of the gains. Reward yourself for your successes. Learn from your setbacks.

One of the universal strategies that enables us to feel more comfortable in the reality of our lives is the presence of support: the people, or whatever there is in our lives that provides us with the comfort, encouragement, affirmation and advice that sustains and replenishes us. The extent to which we develop and use a support system is partly determined by our attitude to support. For some people it may have negative associations with weakness, inadequacy or being smothered, while for others support is seen as an enabling, strengthening presence. A supportive relationship is a great resource, but it is unreasonable to expect one person to meet all of our needs. The challenge is to develop and maintain a number of supportive relationships. We may, for example, unload a lot of our work frustrations on to a partner or a close friend when what we need is the support of a trusted colleague who knows our work and can stand with us non-judgementally in our frustrations and joys. Staff support groups can usefully meet this need. Of course, the best care teams *are* supportive to each other, but it can be helpful to set aside a specific time each week for the team to review their work, share satisfactions and frustrations, learn from each other's experience and to team-build.

Clearly, it is not just from other people that support comes. We can support ourselves through valuing ourselves, nurturing ourselves and through our beliefs. Supporting ourselves is a key element in managing ourselves well, so that we can live and work more effectively.

Some strategies for managing stress

- Develop your problem-solving skills. People tend to deny, ignore or muddle through problems with a consequent increase in stress. Confront the problem, explore the issues, decide on some ways forward, take the first step.
- Develop your assertiveness skills. Considerable stress can be caused by not being able to express your needs, put your point of view, make requests, say no. Be aware of your body/voice. Does it 'collapse' when you make requests or express your needs? Where do your eyes go? Stay relaxed. Get the person's attention. Be specific and concise. Be persistent. Stay in the same gear (don't get irritated or defeated). Give feedback ('Thank you for your time. This is important to me.'). Remember assertiveness is not aggressiveness: aggressiveness denies other people their rights and needs, while communicating assertively respects them.

- Be aware of how your thinking about stressful situations adds to your discomfort. Learn to use positive inner speech to challenge negative thoughts. For example, if you find yourself often worrying that you haven't done things right or well enough, ask yourself, 'Is there any evidence for thinking that?' Tell yourself, 'I always do the best I can and my best *is* good enough'. Tell yourself, 'I don't have to be perfect to be valued and accepted'. Be aware of successes, accomplishments and positive outcomes in previous work. Be open to positive feedback from clients and colleagues.
- Notice your breathing. Hyperventilation is a common habit pattern that produces symptoms similar to the stress syndrome. Over-breathing in stress situations exacerbates the symptoms of stress. Slower abdominal breathing quietens and calms the mind and body.
- Learn the art of relaxation. We don't necessarily relax when we sit down to read a book or watch television. Doing a quick 'body check' at these times will raise your awareness of residual tension. Progressive muscle relaxation, the use of relaxing visualization/imagery and meditation can be learnt from books, tapes or classes. Learning The Alexander Technique can help you use your body in a more efficient, less stressed way.
- Nurture yourself: get enough sleep, take care of your nutritional needs, reduce caffeine/alcohol intake, treat yourself to a sauna or massage, take a weekend break, listen to some music, take a bath, 'shower the day off'. Make yourself a favourite meal, put on your most comfortable clothes. Have some time to yourself. Make love. Enjoy your garden or the countryside.
- Have plenty of distractors in your life – conversation, pastimes, interests, exercise. Regular exercise helps by releasing tension, providing a sense of well-being, supporting self-esteem.
- Unburden to a friend or colleague. Talking about a stressful situation helps us to see it more clearly or differently. Having a good shout/cry/swear/ laugh helps unload distress and frees us for the next piece of living. Learning co-counselling is a useful more structured way of doing this within organizations such as the social services or hospitals.
- Artistic expression (art, music, dancing) can facilitate release of stress.
- Develop and maintain a good support system. Relationships are a mutual source of help, advice, encouragement, affirmation.
- Create stability zones and rituals. Build routines and rituals into your day that are sanctuaries from the pressures of everyday life. Taking the dog for a walk, the drive home, pottering in the garden, taking short periods of meditative time out, allowing yourself to be enveloped by a favourite piece of music.

Self-enquiry Box

The pleasure list
  Think of 20 things that give you pleasure and list them. Now think about how often you allow yourself these pleasures – frequently, occasionally, rarely. Think about whether these pleasures are expensive, inexpensive or cost nothing. Finally think about whether you can enjoy these pleasures alone or whether they require company.
  Reflect on your list and how you incorporate pleasure into your life.

Self-enquiry Box

Guided visualization
  Sit quietly for a few minutes. Now imagine yourself walking down a side street in a large city and up ahead you see a building that looks different from all the rest. As you approach, you see above the door a sign which reads 'This Building is Dedicated to Silence. All Are Welcome.' Imagine yourself opening the door and stepping inside. There, in front of you, is a large octagonal room. The room is bathed in soft coloured light from stained glass windows. There are comfortable chairs placed around the room and you find one and sit down. As you sit you there you become aware of an enveloping calm. You become aware of the stillness and peacefulness that surrounds you. Picture yourself sitting comfortably in this quiet peaceful space. Picture yourself relaxed, immersed in this oasis of calm. Allow yourself to be refreshed by the silence that surrounds you. Allow yourself to be restored by the soothing tranquillity that surrounds you.
  When you are ready, imagine yourself unhurriedly getting up, walking out of the room, opening the door and stepping back into the street. Be aware of the calmness, the peacefulness that you are taking with you. Be aware that you can return to this place at any time.

22 Guided reflection on practice

Why bother with supervision? First, supervision is a significant source of support where we can focus on the difficulties, challenges and successes of our work and have our supervisor share some of the responsibility for our work with clients. Second, it forms part of our continuing learning as a professional. As Casement (1985) comments, 'As professionals we are in a process of becoming, that begins, continues, but never ends.' Supervision helps us use our personal resources more effectively, manage our workload better, challenges inappropriate interventions and ways of coping. Finally, good supervision can help reduce stress, prevent burnout and increase job satisfaction (Butterworth and Faugier, 1992).

Self-enquiry Box

Inskipp and Procter (1992) refer to the 'opportunities' that need to exist within an organization for professionals to stay 'competent and creative' in their work with people. These include the opportunity for:

- *Sharing their work with colleagues.*
- *Getting feedback and guidance.*
- *Developing skills, ideas, information.*
- *Acknowledging feelings.*
- *Feeling valued and affirmed professionally (Inskipp and Procter, 1992).*

You may find it helpful reflect on the extent to which these opportunities are available to you in your practice.

Many nurses may feel that some of these opportunities already exist in the working structures and professional development activities that they have access to – training courses, staff meetings, case conferences, casework supervision and more informally in their contact and conversations with colleagues. It is the responsibility of the individual to assess whether and to what extent these needs are being met in their current working environment and, where opportunities are lacking, they may consider more formal supervision a worthwhile option (formal in the sense of being explicit, negotiated and regular).

Realistically, few organizations are likely to provide funding for 'consultancy supervision' from someone outside the organization. Most often it is provided through a line manager or team leader. While this can be a successful and helpful arrangement, it can raise considerable disclosure anxiety, 'Will I be thought of as inadequate? Unable to cope? Overemotional? How will it affect my career development?' While some of these issues will surface in any supervisory relationship, they have more of an edge in a hierarchical organization where the supervisor is in a position of authority over the supervisee. It also raises fundamental questions about the nature of the supervisory relationship which, for trust and a sense of safety to develop, needs to be seen as a collaborative relationship between equals. This may be difficult to achieve unless there is a flattening of the authority pyramid.

It is all too easy to slide into a passive aggrieved state of mind, feeling unsupported with little opportunity for change and development. There is, I believe, a case for health care professionals to be more proactive in getting more of what they need to function more effectively in their professional role. There are a number of options for getting supervision – from group supervision to one-to-one supervision in a peer relationship.

Being proactive starts with what Casement calls 'self-supervision'. In recent years, the term reflective practice has crept into the vocabulary of nursing as a valued criterion of professionalism. Learning from experience begins with the ability to notice and reflect awarely on what happens in our interactions with patients and clients. This is a skill that deepens with practice. Johns (1993) defines professional supervision as 'the milieu in which reflective practice is facilitated'. This process of self-supervision involves asking reflective questions: 'What did I do and say?' 'Why did I intervene as I did?' 'What did the client do and say?' 'What was I feeling?' 'How did the client feel?' 'What was the outcome?' 'What other choices did I have?' 'How do I feel now about the experience?' 'What have I learnt?' This reflection on the process of care can be enhanced if supervisees write-up significant interpersonal events in a log or journal. Additionally, the use of audio recordings of work with clients can provide challenging but insightful material. Reflecting on practice in this way helps identify issues that can be explored and learnt from in supervision.

Being proactive does not stop with setting up some form of supervision. We need to be active in taking our share of responsibility for ensuring we get the supervision we want. This involves negotiating and contracting. It is important that both supervisor and supervisee communicate with each other their view of the purpose of the sessions and explore how far their expectations match, including their initial hopes and fears. Boundaries need to be established by clarifying the frequency and duration of sessions, the sort of issues it is appropriate to bring, the question of confidentiality, managerial requirements and how supervision is to be evaluated.

Supervision for most nurses represents a shift in practice habits and, as with any change, there can be blocks that prevent the desired outcome. The blocks may be internal: the supervisee may feel themselves to be in a vulnerable position – the supervisory relationship, however benign and equal, is always likely to restimulate experiences of previous relationships with authority figures. Dependency issues surface, to which the supervisee may react by surrendering their autonomy or by becoming resistant to feedback and guidance. There are likely to be anxieties about being judged. Supervision can evoke the 'inner critic', threatening to leave the supervisee feeling demoralized and de-skilled. Supervision commonly has connotations, which are false in this context, of being told what to do, of having one's work overseen. Qualified professionals may also feel that their status and competence is detracted from rather than enhanced by having supervision.

The blocks may be also external, related to the organizational context of supervision. The nursing culture places a high value on emotional control and coping behaviour. This is understandable given the nature of the work but, if these attributes are overemphasized, they detract from the humanity of nurses. Jourard (1971) has commented on how the essential fallibility and vulnerability of the person in the professional role can get masked and the 'real self' alienated. This leads to a high level of professional detachment in which the person is hardly visible in the role, which is not conducive to the development of therapeutic relationships. Nurses tend to collude in not recognizing each other's stresses and problems. It seems that nursing as a profession whose business is caring for others is notoriously bad at caring for its own. It may be that many nurses, like other professional helpers, seek out a helping career as a way of dealing with their own unmet needs for care and intimacy, which are then projected on to the client. Helpers need clients, just as clients need helpers. There is nothing wrong in this just so long as it is recognized and not allowed to creep adversely into the transaction between nurse and patient, for example, by the nurse colluding with the patient's helplessness. These complex dynamics can make it difficult for nurses to enter freely into supervision.

As already indicated, the dual role of line manager and supervisor may present problems and create blocks in the supervision process. There may be trust issues – 'how much of myself and my practice can I safely expose to someone whose managerial responsibilities include monitoring and assessing the quality of my work?' Where the managerial task is seen essentially as enabling and the power held is based on relationship and expertise rather than position, then clinical supervision by line managers can be effective. A further issue in managerial supervision is that the supervisee may experience a conflict between the organizational priorities and objectives, for which the manager has responsibility, and their own. A consequence of this can be that the focus of the supervision dialogue becomes restricted or, worse, degenerate into a 'checking ritual' of visits made, strategies implemented and noting of outcomes.

Supervision options
- Regular one-to-one supervision with a team leader/line manager.
- Regular one-to-one supervision with an experienced colleague from another discipline.
- Regular one-to-one supervision with an 'consultant' from outside the organization.
- Regular one-to-one supervision with a peer (sharing time equally in role of supervisor/supervisee).
- Group or team supervision with clinical team leader or outside 'consultant' as supervisor.

The role of supervisor

Many different grades of staff find themselves in a supervisory role. Senior practitioners, service managers, team leaders, nurse teachers are examples. Given the misconceptions that exist about the role of the supervisor, it is important that supervisors of clinical and casework practice are clear about the role a supervisor plays and are adequately prepared. Part of that preparation is to be aware of underlying needs and issues that the supervisor may seek to meet through the supervisory relationship to the detriment of the process as a learning experience for the supervisee. For instance, the need for power or affirmation may be expressed in the supervisory relationship by the supervisor adopting a guru-like status. Vertical relationships in strongly hierarchical and patriarchal organizations, such as hospitals and community health care services, do not lend themselves to relationships in which collaboration on a basis of equality and mutual respect for the other's professional autonomy can easily flourish. As Johns identifies, there needs to be a shift in the emphasis of the manager's role from delegator and supervisor of work to enabler. A similar shift in emphasis would apply to the nurse teacher engaged in supervision – in this case from didactic teacher to facilitator of student-centred learning.

The key to good supervision is the relationship between supervisor and supervisee. In that sense it is analogous to the helper/client relationship and, just as in the psychotherapeutic alliance the relationship is part of the therapy, so in a similar way the relationship in supervision is a key learning opportunity. The supervisee learns about enabling relationships through being in one. It needs to be stressed, however that, while the relationship may mirror the therapeutic alliance, the focus of the relationship is educational rather than therapeutic. Clearly, personal issues arising out of the supervisee's work experience, which have a bearing on their professional effectiveness, will quite legitimately sometimes be a focus for the supervision dialogue. There is, however, a danger that the supervisee may be filling an unacknowledged need for counselling. Equally, the supervisor may be acting out a need to demonstrate their therapeutic skill or to prove their worth. In this scenario, supervision would unhelpfully become more like therapy.

Butterworth and Faugier suggest the role and function of the supervisor is to encourage personal and educational growth and provide support for clinical autonomy. Hawkins and Shoet see the supervisor's role as a synthesis of education, support and management.

The educative function of supervision is concerned with developing the skills and understandings of the supervisee. This can be achieved through a process of guided reflection on their work with clients and patients (Temple, 1991). Through this exploration the supervisee gathers insights into the dynamics of their interaction with clients. They can explore the meaning of the client's behaviour and the meaning the client's behaviour has for them: how they intervened; the outcomes of that intervention; and alternative ways of responding to this and similar client behaviour. This is not a process in which the task of supervisor is to be the all-knowing expert. While interpretation and guidance from the supervisor may be valued and helpful, the primary task of the supervisor is to facilitate critical thinking. Didactic and prescriptive supervision may lead to what Schon (1991) refers to as a 'learning bind' in which both the educator and learner adopt stances which impede professional growth: 'an open dialogue in which the learner's experience and intuitive knowing is valued fails to develop and the learner feels in awe of the educator's mastery and expertise'. It can be helpful if supervisors are prepared to acknowledge openly their own puzzlement. As Lidmilla (1992) comments, 'If the supervisor can accept his own puzzlement it will help practitioners accept their own limitations without feeling inadequate simply because they are confused about a client's behaviour or have made an intervention error'.

The supportive function of the supervisor is concerned with helping the supervisee to take care of him or herself. Nursing is emotional work. Feelings arise through empathizing with the client, through encountering clients whose experience contain echoes of their own past or present, or simply through a direct reaction to the human anguish that is part of the experience of health care. While feelings often have to be put on one side in order to function effectively, not attending to those feelings leads to the development of defensive strategies for staying distant from patients, the accumulation of stress and ultimately to burnout. Smith (1992), in her study of the 'emotional labour of nursing', concludes that nurses are better able to care for patients when they felt cared for themselves by trained staff and teachers. Faugier (1992), in identifying some of the characteristics of the effective supervisor, comments on the need for him/her to be open to and able to stay with the feelings the supervisee brings. The culture of nursing has traditionally been non-cathartic with emotional control and coping being excessively valued. Bringing personal feelings into the supervision dialogue can be threatening if a 'safe base' has not been established in the form of a relationship of trust. Anxieties about being seen as overemotional, overinvolved, unable to cope or being thought a wimp may surface. It is important that supervisors are able to promote the view that an acknowledgement of feelings is both a strength and a constituent part of good practice in the human relations dimension of health care. We cannot treat people with sensitivity and care if we deny our own humanity.

The managerial function is concerned primarily with quality assurance. Many supervisors will have a responsibility to their organization for the delivery of effective and ethical care and meet that responsibility through the supervision of practitioners' case loads. This many involve looking at assessment data, care plans, strategies and progress notes. There is a responsibility to respond to unsafe and unethical practice and to temper therapeutic idealism with realistic optimism. However, the main task is to collaborate with the supervisee in reviewing their performance with the intention of enabling the practitioner to provide therapeutic care of a high standard. There may be some conflict of interest between the practitioner's ideas and aspirations and the organization's vision of the service that can be provided. This conflict will need to be addressed and managed if the practitioner is to stay committed to the work and not become cynical and disillusioned.

As has been emphasized, it is the relationship that is the key to good supervision. A number of writers, for example Hawkins and Shoet (1989), Reynolds (1990) and Faugier (1992), have commented that the skills and characteristics that supervisors need are similar to those required for counselling. Many identify characteristics that are akin to the 'core conditions for effective helping' (empathy, congruence, openness, genuineness, respect, warmth, acceptance) developed by Carl Rogers in his extensive writing and in his therapeutic and educational work (Kirschenbaum and Henderson, 1990). It would seem important that the supervisor is able to communicate these qualities in their work with practitioners for the unfolding of personal and professional potential to take place.

Heron's interpersonal skills model, Six Category Intervention Analysis (1990) has value as a framework for developing a supervision dialogue. The model identifies a cluster of skills, which have a common intention and are accordingly grouped into one of six categories.

- Catalytic interventions, including active listening skills, questioning and reflective responses, are concerned with eliciting self-discovery talk.
- Challenging interventions may involve giving feedback, correcting or disagreeing, playing 'devil's advocate' and asking confronting questions. They are concerned with raising the supervisee's awareness of blind spots, such as unhelpful patterns of behaviour, thinking errors, deficiencies and strengths, unsafe or unwise practice and successes.
- Supportive interventions will have the intention to validate and affirm the supervisee and their work.
- Cathartic interventions, such as 'giving permission', empathic respond-ing, literal description, the judicious use of touch and proximity and re-enactment, are intended to assist the supervisee to verbalize and discharge feelings appropriately and safely. They may help the practitioner go into unacknowledged feelings being held on the edge of awareness which are relevant to the issues being discussed. Heron makes the important point that suppressed feelings act as a screen preventing us from seeing a situa-tion as clearly as we might, or from a different perspective. In addition, they will trap energy which would otherwise be free for problem solving. Hence new insights and understandings are likely to emerge from cathartic work.
- Informative interventions are concerned with providing information and interpretations relevant to the needs and interests of the supervisee. As has been noted earlier, when this is overdone it impedes the development of critical thinking and the growth of professional confidence and auton-omy. On the other hand, if it is underdone, this can hold the supervisee in a disempowered state.
- Prescriptive interventions are ways of responding that assist the super-visee find the way forward. The supervisor collaborates in a process of creative problem solving and suggesting alternative ways of managing problems presented by the client or patient. As Heron points out, the style in which prescriptive interventions are made follows a continuum from consultative at one end to authoritative at the other. With this in mind, it is important that supervision does not perpetuate what Lidmilla (1992) refers to as the infantile fantasy of 'omnipotent narcissism in the supervisor and idealisation in the supervisee'.

The narrative accounts of our work that we share in supervision are often problem laden. The problem is commonly located within ourselves as prac-titioners, rather than the relationship or the organizational context, and lead to conclusions of inadequacy or failure. According to White (1997) the narrative accounts that are shared are often 'thin' descriptions of practice and seldom represent the richness of a practitioner's work. He argues that supervision can be seen as a re-authoring conversation in which 'negative truths' about practice can be deconstructed.

There are times when our work as mental health nurses seems hardly worthwhile. When it seems to achieve little. When the client seems 'lost' to their illness or retreats behind a wall of resistance and refuses to engage in the helping/healing process. There are times when the experiences of people seeking help seem crushing and insurmountable. There are times when we feel drained with seemingly nothing left to give. It is because the helping relationship can be so depleting that good supervision has such a vital role to play in replenishing practitioners and maintaining effective and innovative practice. Supervision offers what Hawkins and Shoet refer to as a 'therapeutic triad' between client, practitioner and supervisor, within which the emotional challenge of helping can be survived, reflected upon and learnt from.

Self-enquiry Box

Figure 22.1 outlines one way of thinking about the factors that influence our performance as practitioners. Consider which quadrant best reflects your experience. How might your supervision help change that experience?

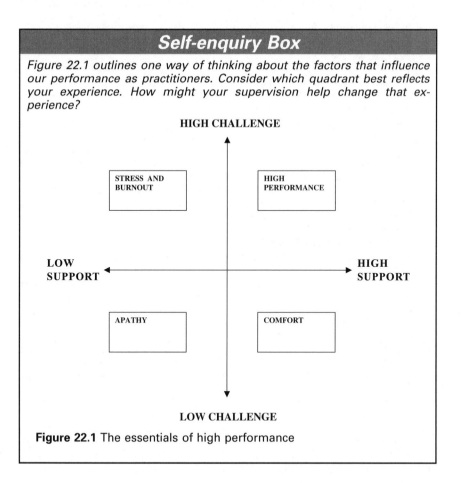

Figure 22.1 The essentials of high performance

References

Ahmed T., Webb Johnson A. (1995) Voluntary groups. In Fernando S. (ed.) *Mental Health in a Multi-Ethnic Society*. London: Routledge.

Ainsworth M. (1991) Attachments and other affectional bonds across the life cycle. In Parkes C. *et al.* (eds) *Attachment Across the Life Cycle*. London: Tavistock/ Routledge.

Argyle M. (1994) *The Psychology of Interpersonal Behaviour*. London: Penguin.

Arnold L. (1995) *Women and Self-Injury – A Survey of 76 Women*. Bristol: Crisis Service for Women.

Atkinson J., Cola D. (1995) *Families Coping with Schizophrenia: A Practitioners Guide to Family Groups*. Chichester: John Wiley & Sons.

Barham P., Hayward R. (1995) *Relocating Madness. From the Mental Patient to the Person*. London: Free Association Books.

Barker P., Reynolds W., Stevenson C. (1997) The human science basis of psychiatric nursing, theory and practice. *Journal of Advanced Nursing*, **25,** 660–667.

Barker P. *et al.* (1998) The wounded healer and the myth of mental wellbeing: ethical issues concerning the mental health status of psychiatric nurses. In Barker P., Davidson B. (eds) *Ethical Strife*. London: Arnold.

Barrowclough C., Tarrier N. (1997) *Families of Schizophenic Patients. Cognitive Behavioural Interventions*. Cheltenham: Stanley Thorn.

Beeforth M., Conlon E., Grayley R. (1994) *Have I Got Views For You*. London: Sainsbury Centre.

Bentall R. (1990) *Reconstructing Schizophrenia*. London: Routledge.

Birchwood M., Tarrier N. (1994) *Psychological Management of Schizophrenia*. Chichester: John Wiley.

Birchwood M., MacMillan F., Smith J. (1994) Early intervention. In Birchwood M., Tarrier N. (eds) *Psychological Management of Schizophrenia*. Chichester: John Wiley.

Borzarth J. (1993) Not necessarily necessary. In Brazier D. (ed.) *Beyond Carl Rogers*. London: Constable.

Bowlby J. (1969) *Attachment and Loss*: Vol. 1 Attachment (2nd edn 1982). London: Hogarth.

Bowlby J. (1973) *Attachment and Loss*: Vol. 2 Separation, Anxiety and Anger. London: Hogarth.

Bowlby J. (1980) *Attachment and Loss*: Vol. 3 Loss, Sadness and Depression. London: Hogarth.

Bowlby J. (1988) A Secure Base. Clinical Applications of Attachment Theory. London: Routledge.

Boyle M. (1990) *Schizophrenia. A Scientific Delusion*? London: Routledge

Brandon D. (1976) *Zen in the Art of Helping*. London: Routledge.

Brandon D. (1991) *Innovation without Change? Consumer Power in Psychiatric Services.* London: Macmillan.

Brandon D. (1997) *The Trick of Being Ordinary.* Cambridge: Anglia Polytechnic University.

Breggin P. (1993) *Toxic Psychiatry.* London: Harper Collins.

Breggin P. (1996) Spearheading a transformation. In Breggin P., Stern M. (eds) *Psychosocial Approaches to Deeply Disturbed Persons.* New York: Haworth Press Inc.

Brown D., Pedder J. (1991) *Introduction to Psychotherapy. An Outline of Psychodynamic Principles in Practice.* London: Routledge.

Brown G. (1996) Life events, loss and depressive disorders. In Heller T. *et al.* (eds) *Mental Health Matters.* Basingstoke: Macmillan.

Burnard P. (1990) *Learning Human Skills. An Experiential Guide for Nurses.* Oxford: Butterworth-Heinemann.

Burns T., Beardsmore A., Bhat A., Oliver A., Mathews C. (1993) A controlled trial of home based acute psychiatric services (1): clinical and social outcomes. *British Journal of Psychiatry,* **163**, 49–54.

Butterworth T., Faugier J. (1992) *Clinical Supervision & Mentorship in Nursing.* London: Chapman & Hall.

Byng-Hall J. (1995) *Rewriting Family Scripts.* New York: Guildford Press.

Campbell P. (1996a) Working with service users. In Sandford T., Gourney K. (eds) *Perspectives in Mental Health Nursing.* London: Bailliere Tindall.

Campbell P. (1996b) *Speaking Our Minds.* Buckingham. Open University Press.

Campbell P., Lindow V. (1997) *Changing Practice. Mental Health Nursing and User Empowerment.* London: Royal College of Nursing.

Caplan G. (1964) *Principles of Preventative Psychiatry.* London: Tavistock.

Casement P. (1985) *On Learning from the Patient.* London: Tavistock Publications.

Chadwick, P. (1996) From a symptom model to a person model. In Chadwick, P., Birchwood, M., Trower, P. (eds) *Cognitive Therapy for Delusions, Voices and Paranoia.* Chichester: John Wiley & Sons.

Chadwick P., Birchwood M., Trower P. (1996) *Cognitive Therapy for Delusions, Voices and Paranoia.* Chichester: John Wiley & Sons.

Clarkson P. (1989) *Gestalt Counselling in Action.* London: Sage Publications.

Clarkson P. (1993) *On Psychotherapy.* London: Whurr Publications.

Clarkson P. (1995) *The Therapeutic Relationship.* London: Whurr Publications.

Coleman R. (1998) *Politics of the Madhouse.* Runcorn: Handsell Publishing.

Conlon E., Gell, C., Grayley, R. *et al.* (1996) *Advocacy A Code of Practice.* London: Department of Health.

Connelly L., Keele, B., Klienbeck, S. *et al.* (1993) A place to be yourself: empowerment from the client's perspective. *Image: Journal of Nursing Scholarship,* **25**, 4.

Copsey N. (1997) *Keeping Faith. The Provision Of Community Mental Health Services Within A Multi Faith Context.* London: Sainsbury Centre for Mental Health.

Cormack D. (1976) *Psychiatric Nursing Observed.* London: Royal College of Nursing.

Davidson B. (1998) The role of the psychiatric nurse. In Barker P., Davidson B. (eds) *Psychiatric Nursing. Ethical Strife.* London, Arnold.

Davidson L., Strauss J. (1992) Sense of self in recovery from severe mental illness. *British Journal of Medical Psychology,* **65**, 131–145.

Davis A., Wainwright J. (1996) Poverty, work and the mental health services. *Breakthrough,* **1**, (1) 47–55.

Davis H., Fallowfield L. (eds) (1991) *Counselling and Communication in Health Care.* Chichester: Wiley.

Dean C., Gadd E. (1990) Home treatment for acute psychiatric illness. *British Medical Journal,* **301**, 1021–1023.

Deegan P. (1988) Recovery: the lived experience of rehabilitation. *Psychosocial Rehabilitation Journal*, **11** (4), 12–19.

Deegan P. (1992) The independent living movement and people with psychiatric disabilities: taking back control over our own lives. *Psychosocial Rehabilitation Journal*, **15** (3), 4–19.

Deegan P. (1995) Recovery as a journey of the heart. *Psychiatric and Rehabilitation Journal*, **19** (5), 91–95.

Deegan P. (1997) Recovery empowerment for people with psychiatric disabilities. *Social Work in Health Care*, **25** (3), 1–24.

De Girolamo G. (1996) W.H.O. studies of schizophrenia: an overview of results & their implications for an understanding of the disorder. In *Department of Health and Home Office (1992) Review Of Health And Social Services For Mentally Disordered Offenders And Others Requiring Similar Services: Services For People From Black and Ethnic Minority Groups; Issues Of Race And Culture. A Discussion Paper*. London: DoH/Home Office.

Department of Health (1990) *Community Care In The Next Decade And Beyond*. London: HMSO.

Department of Health (1994) *Working In Partnership: A Collaborative Approach To Care*. London: HMSO.

Department of Health (1999) *National Service Frameworks for Mental Health. Modern Standards and Service Models*. London. HMSO.

Dupont-Joshua A. (1996) Race, culture and the therapeutic relationship: working with difference creatively. *Counselling*, August.

Dyson J., Cobb M., Forman D. (1997) The meaning of spirituality: a literature review. *Journal of Advanced Nursing*, **26**, 1183–1188.

Egan G. (1994) *The Skilled Helper. A Problem Management Approach To Helping*. Pacific Grove: Brooks Cole.

Fadden G., Kuippers L., Bebbington P. (1987) The burden of care: the impact of functional psychiatric illness on the patient's family. *British Journal of Psychiatry*, **150**, 285–292.

Faugier J. (1992) The supervisory relationship. In Butterworth C., Faugier J. (eds) *Clinical Supervision and Mentorship in Nursing*. London: Chapman & Hall.

Fernando S. (1995) Social realities and mental health. In Fernando S. (ed.) *Mental Health in a Multi-ethnic Society*. London: Routledge.

Fisher D. (1999) A new vision of recovery. *National Empowerment Centre Newsletter*. Spring.

Ford R., Ryan P. (1997) Labour intensive. How effective is intensive support for people with long standing mental illness. *Health Service Journal*, 23rd January.

Fromm E. (1993) *The Art of Being*. London: Constable.

Gallop R. (1998) Abuse of power in the nurse client relationship. *Nursing Standard*, **12** (37), 43–47.

Gergen K. (1990) Therapeutic professionals and the diffusion of deficit. *Journal of Mind and Behaviour*, **11**, 353–368.

Gersie A. (1991) *Storymaking In Bereavement*. London: Jessica Kingsley Publishers.

Gibson L. (1991) A concept analysis of empowerment. *Journal of Advanced Nursing*, **16**, 354–361.

Goldberg, D. Huxley, P. (1992) *Common Mental Disorders: A Bio-social Model*. London: Tavistock.

Gomm R. (1996) Mental health & inequality. In Heller T. *et al* (ed.) *Mental Health Matters*. Basingstoke: Macmillan.

Goodman L., Ross M., Russo N. (1993) Violence against women: physical and mental health effects. Part 1: Research findings. *Applied and Preventative Psychology*, **2**, 77–89.

Gournay K. (1996) Case management. In Sandford T., Gourney K. (eds) *Perspectives In Mental Health Nursing*. London: Baillière Tindall.

Griffiths P., Leach G. (1998) Psychosocial nursing: a model learnt from experience. In Barnes E. *et al.* (eds) *Face to Face with Distress*: Oxford: Butterworth-Heinemann.

Groves P. (1998) Doing and being: a Buddhist perspective on craving and addiction. In Barker P., Davidson B. (eds) *Ethical Strife*. London: Arnold.

Hargie O., Saunders C., Dickson D. (1994) *Social Skills in Interpersonal Communication*. London: Routledge.

Harrison G. (1997) Risk assessment in a climate of litigation. *British Journal of Psychiatry*, **170** (suppl. 32), 37–39.

Hawkins P., Shoet R. (1989) *Supervision in the Helping Relationship*. Buckingham: Open University Press.

Heron J. (1990) *Helping The Client. A Creative And Practical Guide*. London: Sage Publications.

Hill R., Hardy P., Sheppard G. (1996) *Perspectives on Manic Depression*. London: Sainsbury Centre For Mental Health.

Holdstock L. (1993) Can we afford not to revise the person-centred concept of self. In Brazier D. (ed.) *Beyond Carl Rogers*. London: Constable.

Holland S. (1995) Interaction in women's mental health and neighbourhood development. In Fernando S. (ed.) *Mental Health in a Multi-ethnic Society*. London: Routledge.

Hopton J. (1997) Towards anti-oppressive practice in mental health nursing. *British Journal of Nursing*, **6**, (15) 874–878.

Horsfall J. (1997) Psychiatric nursing. Epistemological contradictions. *Advances in Nursing Science*, **20** (1), 56–65.

Inglesby E. (1998) Creating from chaos. In Barker P., Davidson B. *Ethical Strife*. London: Arnold.

Illich I. (1977) *Limits To Medicine*. London: Penguin.

Inskipp F., Proctor B. (1992) *Skills for Supervising & Being Supervised (Audiotape)*. Hastings: Alexia Publications.

Jackson S., Stevenson C. (1998) The gift of time from the friendly professional. *Nursing Standard*, **12** (51), 31–33.

Johns C. (1993) Professional supervision. *Journal of Nursing Management*, **I**, 9–18.

Josselyn (1987) *Finding Herself: pathways to identity development in women*. London: Jossey–Bass.

Jourard S. (1971) *The Transparent Self*. London: Van Nostrand Reinhold Company.

Kanter J. (1985) Case management of the young adult chronic patient: a clinical perspective. *New Directions for Mental Health Services*, **27**, 77–92.

Kirschenbaum H., Henderson V. (1990) *The Carl Rogers Reader*. London: Constable.

Knowles M. (1991) *The Adult Learner: a Neglected Species*. London: Gulf Publishing.

Kuipers L. (1991) Schizophrenia and the family. *International Review of Psychiatry*, **3**, 105–117.

Kuipers L., Leff J., Lam D. (1992) *Family Work for Schizophrenia. A Practical Guide*. London. Gaskell /Royal College of Psychiatrists.

Leete E. (1987) The treatment of schizophrenia: a patient's perspective. *Hospital and Community Psychology*, **38**, 486.

Leff J., Kuippers L., Berkowitz R., *et al.* (1982) A controlled trial of intervention in the families of schizophrenic patients. *British Journal of Psychiatry*, **141**, 121–134.

Leff J., Kuippers L., Berkowitz R., Sturgeon D. (1985) A controlled trial of intervention in the families of schizophrenic patients: two-year follow up. *British Journal of Psychiatry*, **146**, 594–600.

Lidmilla A. (1992) The way of supervision. *Counselling*, May, 97–100.

Lietner (1993) Authenticity, congruence and transparency. In Brazier D. (ed.) *Beyond Carl Rogers*. London: Constable.

Lynch G. (1997) Words and silence. Counselling and psychotherapy after Wittgenstein. *Counselling*, May, 126–128.

Marks I., Connelly J., Muijen M. (1994) Home based versus hospital based care for people with severe mental illness. *British Journal of Psychiatry*, **165**, 179–194.

Maslow A. (1954) *Motivation and Personality*. New York: Harper and Row.

Mason W., Breen D., Marsh I. (1994) Solution focused therapy and in patient psychiatric nursing. Journal of Psycho-Social Nursing, **32** (10), 46–49.

Masson J. (1988) *Against Therapy*. London: Fontana.

McCleod J. (ed.) (1998) The politics of counselling. *In An Introduction to Counselling*. Buckingham: Open University Press.

McDermott G. (1998) Relapse: helping clients to recognise early signs. *Mental Health Nursing*, **18** (6), 22–23.

McDougall T. (1997) Patient empowerment: fact or fiction? *Mental Health Nursing*, **17** (1), 4–5.

Mearns D., Thorne B. (1999) *Person Centred Counselling in Action*. London: Sage Publications.

Mental Health Act Commission (1997) *The National Visit: A One Day Visit to 309 Acute Psychiatric Wards*. London: HMSO.

Mental Health Foundation (1997) *Knowing Our Own Minds. A Survey Of How People in Emotional Distress Take Control of their Lives*. London: MHF.

Mental Health Foundation Briefing (1997) *Mental Health and Housing*. London: Mental Health Foundation.

Miller A. (1990) *The Drama of Being a Child*. London: Virago.

MIND (1993) *Policy On Black And Minority Ethnic People and Mental Health*. London: MIND Publications.

Minghella E., Ford, R., Freeman, T. *et al.* (1998) *Open All Hours: 24-hour Response to People with Mental Health Emergencies*. London: Sainsbury Centre for Mental Health.

Moore C. (1996) *The Re-enchantment of Everyday Life*. London: Hodder & Stoughton.

Morgan S. (1993) *Community Mental Health: Practical Approaches to Long Term Problems*. London: Chapman & Hall.

Morgan S. (1996) *Helping Relationships in Mental Health*. London: Chapman & Hall.

Morgan S. (1998) *Assessing and Managing Risk*. Brighton: Pavillion Publishing Ltd.

Morgan S., Hemming M. (1999) Balancing care and control: risk management and compulsory community treatment. *Mental Health Care*, **3** (1), 19–21.

Mosher B. and Burti, L. (1994) *Community Mental Health*. London: W.W. Norton.

Onyett S. (1998) *Case Management in Mental Health*. Cheltenham: Stanley Thorn.

Nehring J., Hill R., Poole L. (1993) *Work, Empowerment and Community. Opportunities for People with Long Term Mental Health Problems*. London: Research and Development in Psychiatry.

Nolan P., Crawford P. (1997) Towards a rhetoric of spirituality in mental health care. *Journal of Advanced Nursing*, **26**, 289–294.

Peplau H. (1988) *Interpersonal Relations in Nursing*. Basingstoke: Macmillan.

Perkins R., Repper J. (1996) *Working Alongside People with Long Term. Mental Health Problems*. London: Chapman & Hall.

Perry C. (1991) *Listen To The Voice Within*. London: SPCK.

Phillips A. (1988) *Winnicott*. London: Fontana.

Philo G. (1997) Dishing out distress. *Open Mind*, May/June.

Podroll E. (1990) *The Seduction Of Madness*. London: Random Century.

Polusny M., Follette V. (1995) Long term correlates of child sexual abuse: theory and review of empirical literature. *Applied And Preventative Psychology*, **4**, 143–166.

Ram Dass, Gorman C. (1989) *How Can I Help?* London: Rider.

Repper J., and Sayce, L. (1997) *Tall Stories from the Backyard: a Survey of 'Nimby' Opposition to Community Mental Health Facilities Experienced by Key Service Providers in England & Wales*. London: MIND.

Repper J., Ford R., Cooke A. (1994) How can nurses build trusting relationships with people who have severe and long term mental health problems? *Journal of Advanced Nursing*, **19**, 1096–1104.

Reynold W., Cormack D. (1990) *Psychiatric and Mental Health Nursing*. London: Chapman & Hall.

Reynolds W. (1990) Teaching Psychiatric and Mental Health Nursing. In: Reynolds W., Cormack D. (eds) Psychiatric and Mental Health Nursing. London: Chapman Hall.

Richardson A., Unell J., Aston B. (1989) *A New Deal for Carers*. London. Kings Fund.

Richie J., Dick D., Lingham R. (1994) *The Report of the Inquiry into the Care and Treatment of Christopher Clunis*. London: HMSO.

Rogers A., Pilgrim D. (1994) Service users' views on psychiatric nurses. *British Journal of Nursing*, **3** (1), 16–18.

Rogers C. (1967) *On Becoming a Person*. London: Constable.

Rogers C. (1977) The Politics of the helping professions. In Kirschenbaum H., Henderson V. (1990) *The Carl Rogers Reader*. London: Constable.

Rogers C. (1978) Do we need a reality. In Kirschenbaum H., Henderson V. (1990) *The Carl Rogers Reader*. London: Constable.

Rogers C. (1980) *A Way of Being*. Boston: Houghton Mifflin.

Rogers C. (1986a) A client centred/person centred approach to therapy. In Kirschenbaum H. and Henderson, V. (ed.) *The Carl Rogers Reader*. London: Constable.

Rogers C. (1986b) Reflections on feelings and transference. In Kirschenbaum H. and Henderson, V. (ed.) *The Carl Rogers Reader*. London: Constable.

Kirschenbaum H., Henderson V. (1990) *The Carl Rogers Reader*. London: Constable.

Rogers C., Freiberg H.J. (1994) *Freedom to Learn*, 3rd edn. New York: Merrill.

Romme M. (1998) *Understanding Voices. Coping With Auditory Hallucinations and Confusing Realities*. Runcorn: Handsell Publications.

Romme M., Escher S. (1993) *Accepting Voices*. London: MIND Publications.

Rose D., Ford, R., Lindley, P. *et al.* (1998) *In Our Experience*. London: Sainsbury Centre.

Rowe D. (1996) *Depression. The Way Out of Your Prison*. London: Routledge.

Royal College of Nursing (1996) *Race, Ethnicity and Mental Health. The Nurse's Responsibility*. London: Royal College of Nursing.

Ryan P., Ford R., Clifford P. (1991) *Case Management and Community Care*. London: Research and Development for Psychiatry.

Sainsbury Centre (1998a) *Keys to Engagement. Review of Care for People with Severe Mental Illness who are Hard to Engage with Services*. London: Sainsbury Centre for Mental Health.

Sainsbury Centre (1998b) *Acute Problems: a Survey of the Quality of Care in Acute Psychiatric Wards*. London: Sainsbury Centre for Mental Health.

Sainsbury Centre (1998c) Pulling together. The role and training of mental health staff. London: Sainsbury Centre for Mental Health.

Santa-Maria C. (1998) Professional burnout. *Breakthrough*, **2** (2), 21–31.

Sasson M., Lindlow V. (1995) Consulting and empowering black mental health system users. In Fernando S. (ed.) *Mental Health in a Multi-ethnic Society*. London: Routledge.

Schon D. (1991) *The Reflective Practitioner*. London: Basic Books.

Seligman M. (1975) *Helplessness: On Depression, Development And Health*. San Francisco: Freeman.

Sheehy G. (1997) *New Passages. Predictable Crises of Adult Life.* London: Harper Collins.

Sheppard M. (1993) Client satisfaction, extended intervention and interpersonal skills in community mental health. *Journal of Advanced Nursing,* **18**, 246–259.

Sherman P., Porter R. (1991) Mental health consumers as case management aides. *Hospital and Community Psychiatry,* **42**, 94–98.

Showalter E. (1987) *The Female Malady: Women, Madness and English Literature 1830–1980.* London: Virago Press.

Skynner R. (1989) *Institutes and How to Survive Them.* London: Routledge.

Smails D. (1998) *Taking Care. An Alternative To Therapy.* London: Constable.

Smith P. (1992) *The Emotional Labour of Nursing.* Basingstoke: Macmillan Education Ltd.

Stewart I., Joines V. (1987) T. A. Today. Nottingham: Lifespace Publishing.

Strathdee G., Thompson K., Carr S. (1997) What service users want from mental health services. In Thompson K. *et al.* (eds) *Mental Health Service Development Skills Workbook.* London: Sainsbury Centre For Mental Health.

Sullivan H.S. (1953) *The Interpersonal Theory of Psychiatry.* New York: W.W. Norton.

Sullivan P. (1998) Therapeutic interaction in mental health nursing. *Nursing Standard,* **12**, (45) 39–42.

Tarrier N., Barrowclough C., Vaughn C., *et al.* (1988) The community management of schizophrenia: a controlled trial of a behavioural intervention with families to reduce relapse. *British Journal of Psychiatry,* **153**, 532–542.

Tarrier N., Barrowclough C., Vaughn C., *et al.* (1989) The community management of schizophrenia: a two-year follow up. *British Journal of Psychiatry,* **154**, 625–628.

Tarrier N., Beckett, R., Harwood, S. *et al.* (1993) A trial of two cognitive behavioural methods of treatment of drug resistant psychotic symptoms in schizophrenic patients: outcomes. *British Journal of Psychiatry,* **162**, 524–532.

Temple A. (1991) Reflection and the charge nurse. *Nursing Standard,* **5** (26), 32–34.

Thomas B. (1997) Management strategies to tackle stress in mental health nursing. *Mental Health Care,* **1** (1), 15–17.

Thorne B. (1992) *Carl Rogers.* London: Sage Publications.

UKCC (1998) *Guidelines for Mental Health and Learning Disability Nursing.* London: United Kingdom Central Council for Nursing, Midwifery and Health Visiting.

UKCC (1999) *Practitioner–Client Relationships and the Prevention of Abuse.* London: United Kingdom Central Council for Nursing Midwifery and Health Visiting.

Usser J. (1991) *Woman's Madness: Misogyny Or Mental Illness?* London: Harvester Wheatsheaf.

Wakelin D. (ed.) (1997) *Needs Assessment and Service Planning. Crisis Point (2).* London: Mental Health Foundation.

Wakelin D. (ed.) (1998) *The Case for Crisis Services. Crisis Point (8).* London: Mental Health Foundation.

Watkins C. (1989) Transference phenomena in counselling situations. In Dryden W. (ed.) *Key Issues for Counselling in Action.* London: Sage Publications.

Watkins P. (1995) *Drama therapy in The Education of Mental Health Professionals.* Dissertation: University of Nottingham.

White M. (1987) Family therapy & schizophrenia. Addressing the 'in the corner' lifestyle. *Dulwich Centre Newsletter* (Dulwich Centre Publications) Spring.

White M. (1997) *Narratives of Therapists' Lives.* Adelaide: Dulwich Centre Publications.

White M., Epston D. (1990) *Narrative Means to Therapeutic Ends.* London: W.W. Norton.

Wilgosh R., Hawkes D., Marsh I. (1994) Solution focused therapy in promoting mental health. *Mental Health Nursing*, **14** (6), 18–24.

Williams J., Watson G. (1996) Mental health that empowers women. In Heller T. *et al.* (ed.) *Mental Health Matters*. Basingstoke: Macmillan.

Winship G. (1995) The unconscious impact of caring for acutely disturbed patients: a perspective for supervision. *Journal of Psychiatric and Mental Health Nursing*, **2**, 227–231.

Wood H. (1994) *Finding a Place – A Review of Mental Health Services for Adults*. London: HMSO.

Index